The

Weight-Inclusive CBT Workbook for Eating Disorders

Tools to Reject Diet Culture, Heal Body Shame & Promote Recovery

LAUREN MUHLHEIM, PSYD | JENNIFER AVERYT, PHD, ABPP | SHANNON PATTERSON, PHD

New Harbinger Publications, Inc.

Publisher's Note

This publication is designed to provide accurate and authoritative information in regard to the subject matter covered. It is sold with the understanding that the publisher is not engaged in rendering psychological, financial, legal, or other professional services. If expert assistance or counseling is needed, the services of a competent professional should be sought.

NEW HARBINGER PUBLICATIONS is a registered trademark of New Harbinger Publications, Inc.

New Harbinger Publications is an employee-owned company.

Copyright © 2026 by Lauren Muhlheim, Jennifer Averyt, Shannon Patterson
New Harbinger Publications, Inc.
5720 Shattuck Avenue
Oakland, CA 94609
www.newharbinger.com

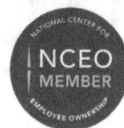

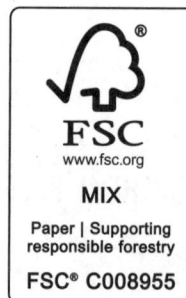

Cover design by Amy Shoup

Acquired by Elizabeth Hollis Hansen

Edited by Karen Levy

Library of Congress Cataloging-in-Publication Data on file

FSC
www.fsc.org
MIX
Paper | Supporting responsible forestry
FSC® C008955

Printed in the United States of America

28   27   26

10   9   8   7   6   5   4   3   2   1   First Printing

"Accessible, affirming, and politically awake, this workbook meets people in the truth of their bodies and their lives. A much-needed tool for those pursuing recovery beyond the narrow frame of thinness and control."

—**Sirius Bonner**, executive leader, cultural strategist, and author of the *Freedom & Desire* Substack

"If you are a clinician or client using enhanced cognitive behavioral therapy (CBT-E), I recommend stopping and ordering *The Weight-Inclusive CBT Workbook for Eating Disorders*. With this workbook, there is no reason to be practicing traditional CBT-E. This workbook is compassionate, accessible, trauma-informed, and takes the weight stigma out of CBT-E. I am excited to add this to the short list of books about eating disorders that I can confidently recommend to colleagues and clients."

—**Rachel Millner, PsyD, CEDS-S, CBTP**

"I wish *The Weight-Inclusive CBT Workbook for Eating Disorders* had existed twenty years ago! Muhlheim, Averyt, and Patterson gently guide the reader through the difficult work of recovering from diet culture. This workbook offers an empowering resource for those seeking peace with body and food, while attending to shame, grief, diverse identities, trauma, and discrimination. This book will be a game changer in the world of self-help for eating disorders."

—**Erin Harrop, PHD, MSW, LICSW**, assistant professor at the University of Denver, and clinician with Opal Food + Body Wisdom

"CBT-WI is a breath of fresh air in a world dominated by weight stigma. The authors have managed to pack in endless amounts of helpful skills and tools while laying out copious evidence that people of all sizes get eating disorders and deserve treatment that is affirming rather than shaming. Thanks to this wonderful workbook, many more people with eating disorders now have a better way forward in their journey toward a durable recovery."

—**Rebecka Peebles, MD, FAAP, DABOM**

"A home run! This welcoming and inclusive workbook presents the key evidence-based strategies of CBT-WI for eating disorders, without the judgment and weight stigma that has plagued our field for too long."

—**Jennifer J. Thomas, PhD**, professor of psychiatry at Harvard Medical School, and codirector of the Eating Disorders Clinical and Research Program at Massachusetts General Hospital

"This groundbreaking cognitive behavioral therapy (CBT) workbook combines evidence-based practices with highly relatable, inclusive, and practical examples and prompts—all of which are (finally!) shared from a weight-inclusive perspective. A wonderful resource!"

—**Jennifer L. Gaudiani, MD, CEDS-C, FAED,** founder and medical director of the Gaudiani Clinic, and author of *Sick Enough*

"Lauren Muhlheim, Jennifer Averyt, and Shannon Patterson have provided a groundbreaking pathway for eating disorder recovery. Combining an evidence-based cognitive behavioral approach with a compassionate appreciation of the power of diet culture, they offer a hopeful and practical way forward. This book will be an invaluable adjunct to therapy for clinicians and clients alike, and for those who are unable to access therapy."

—**Anthea Fursland, PhD**, clinical psychologist

"I have been waiting years for this book to be written. It is exactly what eating disorder clinicians and patients need."

—**Cheri A. Levinson, PhD**, professor at the University of Louisville, director of the Eating Anxiety Treatment (EAT) Lab, and founder of the Louisville Center for Eating Disorders

"This is a beautifully crafted workbook that makes eating disorder recovery more accessible. Free from harmful, weight-centered rhetoric, it provides a genuinely supportive path to healing, and is highly recommended for anyone facing difficulties around food and eating."

—**Sumner Brooks, MPH, RDN,** founder of EDRD Pro, and coauthor of *How to Raise an Intuitive Eater*

"An invaluable addition to the field. Weight-Inclusive CBT (CBT-WI) addresses critical yet often neglected aspects of eating disorder treatment, offering people of all body sizes tools to challenge diet culture and nurture recovery. With its nondiet, all-foods-fit approach, it pushes back against weight bias, stigma, and the pervasive influence of diet culture—making it a must-read for anyone who has ever felt overlooked in eating disorder care, and professionals committed to inclusive, respectful treatment."

—**Suzanne Bailey-Straebler, PhD**, clinical director of the Center for Eating Disorders at Weill Cornell Medicine, and coauthor of *Group Cognitive Behavior Therapy for Eating Disorders*

Contents

Foreword

When it comes to eating disorder treatment, the news is invariably mixed. On the one hand (bad news), eating disorders are notoriously challenging to overcome. On the other hand (good news), years of careful research has produced an evidence-based treatment that works well across the spectrum of problematic eating behaviors; that treatment is cognitive behavioral therapy, or CBT.

Unfortunately (more bad news), many individuals who struggle with eating disorder symptoms simply don't have access to CBT—either with or without the support of a therapist. The reasons for this are myriad, including the fact that access to evidence-based psychotherapy for any disorder is limited, and this is even more true for eating disorders. Another barrier to access is that some therapists who embrace a weight-inclusive approach to eating disorder treatment have started turning away from CBT because existing CBT manuals for eating disorders insufficiently address this perspective. And some clients, particularly those in higher-weight bodies, report having found traditional CBT inadequate in acknowledging their many experiences with discrimination and weight-based stigma, including in health care.

Finally, many CBT self-help resources were written before it was widely acknowledged that eating disorders disrupt the lives of all types of people. As such, these resources typically were not written for those who are minoritized, which means readers have to try to follow the challenging advice in the book (because CBT is hard even under the best of circumstances!), while managing their emotional reactions to well-meaning but ultimately invalidating messaging.

And now for the good news. This book was written with the explicit aim of addressing all the above issues. The authors have sought to increase access and use of CBT by blending very traditional, tried-and-true, evidence-based CBT strategies with a modern, updated inclusive approach aimed at addressing the needs of a much more diverse range of people struggling with eating disorders, including but not limited to those living in larger bodies. As a result, this book has much to offer those who live with eating disorders and those who treat eating disorders.

For those who live with eating disorders, this book can help you help yourself, whether you have a therapist or not. It combines the best that CBT has to offer, including all the important core strategies, combined with years of the authors' collective clinical wisdom and recent research on auxiliary approaches to make sure that you can tailor the CBT strategies as needed. As a long-standing CBT therapist, I was delighted to see so many strategies that I know are crucial to the success of CBT explained in such a clear and inclusive voice.

For those who treat eating disorders, this book can serve both as a supplemental resource that you can give to your clients and as a guide for how to modify traditional CBT in a very thoughtful way to address the needs of the vast array of clients who present with eating disorders. I can also see using this book to validate clients who struggle to accept they have an eating disorder because they don't conform to the incorrect but widely accepted eating disorder stereotype.

We know that eating disorders impact everyone regardless of age, race, ethnicity, gender, ability, or body size; thus, providers need resources that help clients feel seen. I highly recommend therapists read this book to glean new insights into adapting CBT while staying true to core principles and strategies. Whether you already consider yourself a CBT practitioner or not, if you treat eating disorders, this resource should be added to your clinical toolbox.

> —Carolyn Black Becker, PhD, ABPP, coauthor of *Eat Without Fear: Harnessing Science to Confront and Overcome Your Eating Disorder* and *Cognitive-Behavioral Therapy for PTSD: A Case Formulation Approach, Exposure Therapy for Eating Disorders*

Acknowledgments

The case examples in this book are all fictional and derived from our collective work over many years with hundreds of clients. We want to acknowledge all the clients with whom we've worked. Thank you for the opportunity to support and learn from you to provide better, more inclusive care.

We are deeply grateful to many people who supported the writing of this book both directly and indirectly. Thank you to the following people who gave feedback on portions of the manuscript: Beth Lieberman, Shira Rosenbluth Dab, Carly Poynter, Elisha Carcieri, Katerina Rinaldi, Shruti Kinkel-Ram, Shelly Bar, Nicole Leschak, and Kate Krautbauer. Thank you to the many colleagues, especially those with lived experience, who have influenced our thinking.

We are incredibly grateful to Carolyn Becker, Sirius Bonner, Patrilie Hernandez, and Scout Silverstein for providing guidance and sensitivity reads. Thanks to Eric Muhlheim for his arduous editing and Tasnia Tarana for her artwork.

Thank you to Terry Wilson for his mentorship, introducing me (Lauren) to CBT for eating disorders, and graciously encouraging me to modify it. Thank you to Rachel Millner, who helped us plant the seeds for this book over many years of collaboration, and to Ragen Chastain, for tirelessly advocating for weight-inclusive care and inspiring this update.

Thank you to our team at New Harbinger, Elizabeth Hollis Hansen and Madison Davis, for supporting our vision for this book.

Lastly, we are grateful to our spouses—Eric, Jon, and Ethan—for keeping us fed while we wrote. We also appreciate the cuddles and walk-ons by Bowie, Sasha, Freddy, Nelson, Joanie, Mira, Hank, Jasmine, and Penelope.

Introduction

If you're reading this book, you've likely been struggling with your eating habits or body image. Welcome—you've come to the right place! We're glad you're seeking more support with your eating and body image. Maybe you are experiencing cycles of restricting and bingeing. Perhaps you limit your food intake, exercise excessively, or are preoccupied with your eating habits. Maybe your guilty feelings drive you to vomit after you eat what you feel is too much, or you use laxatives to counteract what you've eaten. Perhaps you obsess over counting calories, counting macros, or avoiding certain foods like sugar, gluten, dairy, or red meat. Maybe you feel distressed over what feels like bouts of "emotional eating." Or you might keep trying diet after diet and become confused about how to eat and be in your body in a world that keeps suggesting new ways to perfect it.

We've written this workbook for everyone who needs support with their relationship to food and their bodies. People of all sizes, genders, races, ethnicities, and abilities can benefit from the skills provided. Those with eating disorders and "disorders of dieting," a term coined by our colleague, Deb Burgard, can find healing in these pages. If you have been diagnosed with anorexia nervosa, bulimia nervosa, binge-eating disorder, or other specified feeding or eating disorder (OSFED), this workbook is for you. If you engage in cycles of dieting and then periods of rebound "overeating," engage in excessive exercise and/or "emotional eating," or are preoccupied with your shape or weight, this workbook is also for you. If you've been told you have muscle dysmorphia, atypical anorexia, or orthorexia, this workbook is for you as well. If you have been diagnosed with avoidant/restrictive food intake disorder (ARFID), this may not be the best workbook for you, but aspects may still be applicable, with modifications.

Note: This book is also for you if you have not been diagnosed or do not believe you have a "full-blown" eating disorder. Many people with disordered eating do not think they're sick enough to qualify for help. However, symptoms can progress quickly, and even those who do not meet the full criteria for an eating disorder can experience significant distress.

We understand that despite the messages from society and other health professionals telling you to change your body, your body is not the problem. The true problems are society's obsession with thinness, the associated pressure to conform, and the failure of spaces to accommodate all bodies.

We will never tell anyone in a bigger body to diet or try to change their body. This includes people who are in the biggest of bodies.

If you have been complimented or praised for weight loss and body changes because of your disordered eating, we see you and are sorry that you've had to experience this. We have empathy for you if you've been told to lose weight. We believe that bodies are meant to be diverse and that trying to change your body, including through dieting, only makes eating problems worse. Furthermore, repeated attempts to alter your body's natural size can create more distress. We will use well-researched techniques derived from cognitive behavioral therapy (CBT) to help you stop problematic behaviors, enhance your body image, and cultivate peace with eating. We will also help you advocate for compassionate and size-inclusive care.

Who Are We?

We are three psychologists who were trained in CBT for eating disorders. Collectively, we have helped hundreds of people from diverse backgrounds navigate eating disorders and related body concerns. Each of us has become concerned that the existing library of CBT-based manuals and books assumes that people with eating disorders are all meant to be thin, suggests weight loss for those in bigger bodies, and downplays the importance of external factors—such as societal weight stigma, systemic oppression, and discrimination—on the development of an eating disorder.

Although two of us live in larger bodies, we think it's important to acknowledge that we are white cisgender women who hold numerous advantaged identities. These advantages have afforded us access to multiple resources, including education. In the continual process of unlearning our biases, we rely on the work of those with lived experience in larger bodies and who hold other marginalized identities. Many of these people are featured throughout this book and in the online resources. Please consider supporting their work.

Why This Book?

This workbook is based on CBT, the best-researched and most effective treatment for eating disorders. It is useful for helping people with all types of eating disorders. CBT suggests that thoughts, behaviors, and emotions are closely related and influence one another. It can help you learn more about your relationship with food, shape, and weight, and how these relationships are interconnected.

This workbook introduces a revised CBT for eating disorders, known as Weight-Inclusive CBT (CBT-WI). You might wonder: What exactly does it mean to be "weight-inclusive"? Ragen Chastain's *Weight and Healthcare* August 2022 newsletter defines weight-inclusive care as "care that is created for bodies of all sizes from the ground up, including research, tools, equipment, best practices, etc., practiced by fully fat-affirming health care practitioners." This includes mental health interventions that are explicitly designed for and include people in bodies of *all* sizes.

How Is CBT-WI Different?

You may have heard of CBT for eating disorders. Perhaps you have even tried this approach, but it hasn't been helpful. How will CBT-WI be different?

- Most other CBT-based self-help books for eating disorders are more than twenty years old. They contain stigmatizing language, examples, and activities and fail to incorporate more recent research and advances in the field (Byrne and Fursland 2024). This workbook aims to provide more inclusive materials and examples that better represent the diverse range of individuals who may experience problems with eating behaviors.

- CBT research has primarily involved white, heterosexual, cisgender women. Previous versions of CBT mainly focused on individuals with smaller bodies and included recommendations for weight loss for those with larger bodies. This book aims to include all bodies, acknowledge the societal impact of oppression, and take a non-diet and all-foods-fit approach. It recognizes that eating disorders can occur for anyone regardless of weight, shape, or body size. There are no modifications based on weight or body mass index (BMI).

- This workbook will not include weekly weighing. Focusing on weight may make progress more challenging and is not necessary for improving disordered eating behaviors. You may still need to have your weight and vitals monitored by a medical professional; we just won't have you track your weight.

- We call out the role of diet culture—a societal system that values people based on their appearance, especially their body size and shape—in contributing to and maintaining disordered eating and body shame.

A Note on Language

We deliberately avoid using the terms "overweight" and "obesity" throughout the book. "Overweight" implies that there is a "right weight," and "obesity" is a medicalized term that has been weaponized against larger people. We instead will use the terms "larger-bodied, "in a bigger body," and "fat," which is a descriptive term that has been reclaimed by fat activists much in the same way that "queer" has been reclaimed by the LGBTQ2S+ (lesbian, gay, bisexual, trans, queer, two-spirit, and others) community (Robbins et al. 2025).

Some of the ideas in this book may be very different from what you hear or have learned from mainstream culture and other health care providers. This workbook may initiate a new way of thinking about food, weight, body image—and living.

How to Use This Workbook and When to Seek Help

People with disordered eating will often benefit from working with a team of health care professionals to treat their symptoms. This may include a therapist, dietitian, and medical provider. However, many people with eating disorders do not have access to treatment. Fortunately, CBT is effective as part of structured treatment with a therapist, as guided self-help with a therapist, or as self-help alone. This workbook is based on a new self-help version of CBT-WI designed to be used alone, with a therapist, or with other team members.

If you think that you may have an eating disorder, be aware that many people who experience these problems can have medical complications. This is why anyone with eating disorder symptoms should see a medical provider (Academy for Eating Disorders [AED] 2021). This is especially true if you are at a low weight or even if you are in a larger body and have recently lost a lot of weight. It is important to pursue medical care if you are engaging in self-induced vomiting; using laxatives; or experiencing other symptoms like lightheadedness, chest pain, or vomiting blood. Similarly, if you are experiencing medical symptoms or other mental health concerns, such as self-harm or thoughts of suicide, in addition to your eating disorder, it is strongly recommended that you speak to your medical or mental health professional about your symptoms. We will also include resources for support related to thoughts of suicide in chapter 1.

We encourage you to speak with your health care provider about your specific disordered eating behaviors. Your doctor can recommend lab work and tests that help identify potential medical issues related to your symptoms and recommend ongoing monitoring of weight, vital signs, and lab results as needed. They can also connect you with specialists who can help manage these symptoms while you pursue recovery.

How to Get Started

We have designed this book to be read in order while completing the associated worksheets, many of which can also be found online at http://www.newharbinger.com/56456. We will provide prompts and ask you to reflect on your learning. The exercises will build on one another. It may be tempting to power through the book, but we strongly encourage you to complete no more than one chapter per week or every other week. In chapter 1, we will provide general information about eating disorders and help you better understand whether this book is right for you. In chapters 2 through 6, you will learn strategies to reduce disordered eating behaviors and find the nourishment you need. In chapters 7 through 10, you will explore body image and learn how your concern with weight/shape impacts your overall well-being and behaviors. CBT-WI is designed to help people with many different types of behaviors. We recognize that some material in the book won't be relevant to you. Feel free to move past sections that do not apply.

This book will help you:

- Understand the role that eating behaviors and body concerns are playing in your life.

- Make changes to your eating behaviors.

- Overcome behaviors such as purging, excessive exercise, and calorie-counting.

- Learn to recognize and trust your body's cues to truly eat enough.

- Improve your body appreciation.

- Increase your ability to tolerate distressing feelings and sensations.

- Understand weight stigma and learn how to challenge diet culture.

To get the best results from this workbook, we invite you to prioritize it. We will ask you to reflect on your learning and make gradual changes. But don't worry—we'll break it down into manageable steps!

Chapter 1

What Is an Eating Disorder and Do I Have One?

You may not identify with having an eating disorder. When you think about someone with an eating disorder, who comes to mind? Powerful social narratives—via television, movies, and other media—influence beliefs we have about who struggles with eating. When you don't see your identities, or people who look like you, represented in media coverage and treatment spaces, it can be hard to believe that you may have an eating disorder. You may also have difficulties accessing eating disorder care if you do not fit the stereotype.

We now have a much better understanding of eating disorders than we once did. For many years, eating disorders were believed to affect mainly young, thin, white, affluent women. As a result, treatment and research was directed toward this population. We recognize that eating disorders affect people of all genders, ages, races, ethnicities, body shapes, weights, sexual orientations, and socioeconomic statuses (AED 2015). Most people with eating disorders are *not* in thin bodies (Duncan, Ziobrowski, and Nicol 2017). Conversely, not everyone in a larger body has an eating disorder. Larger bodies are not a symptom or a problem to be explained—they are a valid and natural part of the diversity of humans. This updated understanding requires the modification of treatment manuals and methods.

Eating disorders are not a chosen way to eat. They often begin as an attempt to reduce or cope with trauma, weight stigma, or other forms of discrimination. Members of the LGBTQ2S+ community are at an elevated risk for disordered eating, which may be related to gender minority stress, such as experiences of identity policing, social rejection, and isolation (Brown et al. 2024; Nagata et al. 2025). Research suggests that LGBTQ2S+ youth are three times more likely to have an eating disorder when compared to their heterosexual peers (Parker and Harriger 2020). Transgender college students report experiencing disordered eating at approximately four times the rate of their cisgender classmates (Diemer et al. 2018).

The *Diagnostic and Statistical Manual of Mental Disorders, Fifth Edition, Text Revision* (DSM–5-TR; American Psychiatric Association 2022) identifies four primary eating disorder diagnoses related to concerns about shape and weight, including anorexia nervosa, bulimia nervosa, binge-eating disorder, and other specified feeding or eating disorder (OSFED). We see these disorders as having more similarities than differences. Fairburn (2008), an early developer of CBT for eating disorders, wrote, "What is most striking is how similar they are" (p. 10). He goes on to say that "there is an arbitrariness to the way [the eating disorder diagnoses are] carved up to create the three diagnostic concepts" (p. 10). A related observation is that many people with eating disorders meet the criteria for different disorders over time (Eddy et al. 2008).

We agree. We see the four eating disorders listed above as having a common maintaining factor: dietary restriction or failure to eat adequately. Undereating causes a predictable and significant cluster of experiences and behaviors. Once established, biological processes help maintain them:

- People with anorexia nervosa fear gaining weight. As a result, they eat less than their bodies need and may engage in other behaviors that keep their body weight lower than what is healthy for their body.

- People with binge-eating disorder also fail to eat enough, but a strong survival mechanism drives them to lose control over eating after periods of restriction. This often takes place in "binges": distinct bouts of eating during which they feel out of control and after which they experience guilt or shame.

- People with bulimia nervosa binge when they don't eat enough. They also engage in additional behaviors—such as self-induced vomiting, misuse of laxatives, or excessive exercise—to minimize the impact of binges.

- Those with OSFED do not neatly fall into one of the above categories but experience behaviors encompassing restriction, bingeing, purging, or overexercising in different combinations and at various frequencies.

Further blurring these categories, the weight bias incorporated into the *DSM-5-TR* influences practitioners' diagnoses. For example, anorexia nervosa is reserved for people who are at objectively low weights. The rest of those with anorexia are diagnosed with "atypical anorexia." While this diagnosis technically falls under OSFED, most research suggests it is the same illness as anorexia nervosa and, in practice, is equally as severe, if not more severe, in terms of psychological and medical symptoms (Golden 2023).

Another example: Because of weight stigma and the presumption that people with binge-eating disorder are often bigger, dietary restriction is not a criterion for binge-eating disorder. However, we have yet to see a person with binge-eating disorder who has not been restricting or had a history of restriction and/or weight suppression (a topic we will discuss in more detail in chapter 2).

You may have noticed that your eating disorder symptoms change over time. Many with disordered eating observe that their symptoms are influenced by other difficulties they have, such as post-traumatic stress, depression, or anxiety. We believe that instead of assigning labels and categorizing yourself based solely on behaviors and personal characteristics—including body size—viewing your symptoms on a continuum may be more helpful.

• *Sasha's Story*

Sasha is a thirty-three-year-old woman who seeks medical care from her primary care doctor yearly. Since getting divorced from her partner, Sasha had to take a second job during nights and weekends to make ends meet. As a result of financial stress and less recreational time, she has been unable to socialize with her friends and family. Additionally, she has had less time to grocery shop and prepare meals. It has been challenging to find time to pack meals and snacks, and even more difficult to take breaks to eat during her busy day as a receptionist in a health care system.

With less food and time available during the day and fewer opportunities for social eating with her support system, Sasha found herself restricting the amount she ate. At first, it was unintentional. As a result of her daytime eating restriction, she was ravenous when she got home. Once she started eating, she found it hard to stop. This behavior made Sasha feel physically ill, ashamed, and embarrassed. To compensate for what she'd eaten the night before, Sasha intentionally began skipping breakfast and taking walks during her lunch break instead of eating. As time went on, Sasha was consumed by fears that she was eating too many calories and began avoiding activities she'd previously enjoyed.

During her yearly physical, Sasha's doctor asked if she had any concerns. Sasha shared her worries about binge-eating behaviors, and her provider recommended limiting carbohydrates, a potentially harmful recommendation that made things worse. She was later referred to a therapist and diagnosed with binge-eating disorder. The therapist encouraged Sasha to record her eating, which helped her realize that it was periods of restriction and limited social support that made her vulnerable to binge eating. They worked together to address both factors. After improving her nutrition, including increasing carbohydrates—and adding in more social activities—Sasha's binge-eating behavior dramatically decreased.

Do You Have an Eating Disorder?

If you have not been diagnosed with an eating disorder, you may wonder whether you have one. The first step is to familiarize yourself with some common signs of disordered eating behaviors and think about whether you are experiencing these now or have experienced them in the past. Please note that some of these signs and behaviors may be related to cultural factors, neurodivergence, trauma, or a lack of consistent access to food. If that is the case, these may not be behaviors that you can change.

Eating Disorder Signs	Experiencing Now	Have Experienced in the Past
I think about my eating, weight, or shape frequently.		
Food dominates my life.		
I am preoccupied with a desire to change my body—to lose weight, to become more muscular, etc.		
I try to restrict how much food I eat most of the time.		
I try to follow strict rules about what I eat, how much I eat, and when I eat.		
I try to stay within a certain number of calories during the day.		
I need to track all the food I eat throughout the day.		
I refuse to eat certain types of food.		
I have rituals related to eating, such as eating certain foods first or chewing a certain number of times.		
I feel a loss of control when eating; it's hard to stop once I've started.		
I am compelled to eat things I believe I should not eat.		
I often feel the desire to eat when emotionally upset or stressed.		
I feel guilty after eating.		

Eating Disorder Signs	Experiencing Now	Have Experienced in the Past
I find myself "grazing" or snacking frequently throughout the day.		
I eat unusually large amounts of food in a short period of time.		
I make myself vomit to lose weight or after eating a large amount of food.		
I use laxatives, diuretics, or diet pills to lose weight or after eating large amounts of food.		
I use water, caffeinated beverages, or nicotine to stay full during the day.		
I exercise to make up for eating large amounts of food.		
I force myself to exercise even if I am tired, injured, or do not feel like exercising.		
I feel guilty if I skip a workout or take a day off from exercise.		
I need to track exercise and/or how many calories I burn during the day.		
I try to avoid eating in front of other people.		
I frequently check my weight, appearance in the mirror, or how my clothes fit.		
I frequently compare myself to others or to pictures of myself.		
I feel very distressed about my body appearance, weight, and/or shape.		
I try to avoid looking at my body, or avoid other people seeing my body.		
My sense of self-worth is closely tied to my weight, shape, and body.		

As shown in the previous table, many eating disorder symptoms are related to behaviors to control or reduce body weight, worries about body appearance and size, and loss of control over eating. If you are currently experiencing any of these concerns or have had them in the past, this indicates that you may have a history of disordered eating behaviors. The more signs you are currently experiencing, the more likely you are to benefit from treatment to address these concerns.

It is also important to consider how these symptoms and behaviors impact other areas of your life. The following questions will help you explore this.

Have Eating Disorder Symptoms Impacted Your Life?	Yes	No
Does spending time on weight, shape, and eating interfere with activities or things you enjoy?		
Have others expressed concern about your eating?		
Have your symptoms made it difficult for you to do your work, go to school, or take care of things at home?		
Have you avoided activities or things you enjoy due to your eating or body concerns?		

If you are currently experiencing multiple disordered eating symptoms and answered "yes" to any of the items above, you likely meet the criteria for one of the eating disorders described earlier. If you notice that you only have some of the symptoms described, you may still benefit from this workbook. CBT-WI can help you with milder eating disorder symptoms as well.

Now that you've taken a closer look at eating disorder symptoms and how they impact your life, consider how you might benefit from this workbook.

What are your goals as you work through CBT-WI?

_____

_____

_____

What Caused Your Eating Disorder?

The causes of eating disorders are complex. Presently, we don't know exactly what *causes* someone's eating disorder. Researchers believe that an interplay of biological, psychological, and social factors causes eating disorders. Genetic and environmental risk factors are each thought to play a significant role. Genes set the stage, and the environment and life events influence how they play out. As you review the factors below, consider whether any are relevant to you. Note that we don't need to understand what caused your eating disorder to help you recover. If you are caught in a cycle of disordered eating, it is impacting your health, and CBT-WI can help!

Genetics

Research indicates that genetic factors (believed to be a combination of genes) account for approximately 39 to 74 percent of the risk for eating disorders (Yilmaz, Hardaway, and Bulik 2015). If you cannot identify relatives with eating disorders, this does not mean that your genes did not play a role. Eating disorders have historically not been discussed or disclosed. Additionally, many folks with such problems may not even recognize that their behaviors are disordered.

Have any family members experienced challenges with food? If you cannot think of anyone who has been diagnosed with an eating disorder, are there people in your family who seem preoccupied with food, weight, or body image? Or are there people in your family who have perfectionism, obsessive-compulsive disorder (OCD), or other types of anxiety disorders? These are often linked to some of the same traits that are linked to eating disorders.

_____

_____

_____

History of Dieting

If we were asked to cite a single gateway behavior that most commonly leads to disorders of eating, it would be dieting. Dieting is a significant risk factor for eating disorders (Stice et al. 2017).

Most often, eating disorders develop following a period of restriction or negative energy balance. The restriction does not need to have been deliberate. It can also result from situations such as illness, overtraining for athletics, attempts to be healthier, or changes in eating habits for medical reasons (Brandenburg and Andersen 2007). Interventions like dieting, bariatric surgery, and GLP-1 medications such as semaglutide also create a negative energy deficit. This causes appetite changes that may increase your vulnerability to developing an eating disorder (Bartel et al. 2024). Many people experience rebound binge eating and regain weight, which is the body's protective response to restriction. Others become caught in restrictive behaviors and remain malnourished.

When was the first time you engaged in dieting behavior or were encouraged to diet? What other weight loss attempts have you made?

_____

_____

_____

Societal Ideals

Environmental factors make room for eating disorders to blossom. Our culture overvalues thinness. It hasn't always been this way: In earlier times, being in a larger body was considered desirable and a sign of wealth and good health. Recently, societal pressures to conform to thinness or muscularity have intensified; it's understandable for people to respond to these expectations.

If you have experienced bullying, teasing, discrimination, or the withholding of resources (e.g., love, inclusion, or access to medical care) because of your size, it makes sense that you would internalize the message that being smaller or thinner will keep you safe. Weight stigma is real; there are many indicators that thinner people have access to more advantages and resources. For example, research has shown that fat people are hired less often (Flint et al. 2016) and that fat women earn less than their smaller peers (Li, Chen, and Yao 2021). Even if you have never been in a larger body, it makes sense that the idea could cause anxiety. Trauma and adverse life events can also increase the desire to align with societal ideals. If you are gender diverse or BIPOC (Black, Indigenous, and People of Color), you may have experienced discrimination that made fitting the white ideal of thinness a survival strategy.

Have you ever felt like your body was a problem or didn't fit with societal standards?

_____

_____

Non-Medical Drivers of Health

While factors such as genetics, dieting, and societal ideals play a role in the development of eating disorders, *non-medical drivers of health* also influence a person's risk of developing an eating disorder. These are environmental conditions that affect a person's health outcomes (Centers for Disease Control [CDC] 2024). These factors include the larger systems that shape the quality of our lives such as access to quality health care, education, economic stability, and discrimination. Forces outside our control—such as political systems, economic policies, and capitalism—influence our well-being. They create oppression that can reinforce eating disorder behaviors. Below we define examples of non-medical drivers of health.

FOOD INSECURITY

You may have grown up in a family where caregivers struggled to provide food regularly. Alternatively, you may currently struggle to access enough food for yourself and your family, which may lead to prioritizing others' needs over your own. These experiences—collectively known as "food insecurity"—may contribute to the development of eating challenges. Research has shown that people who experience food insecurity are at higher risk for developing eating disorders (Becker et al. 2019; Burke et al. 2023; Hazzard et al. 2020). Unreliable access to food throughout the month can lead to a binge-restrict cycle that is beyond your direct control. This cycle can trap you, increasing the challenge of recovery from an eating disorder. Our online resources provide ideas to increase access to food in the handout Satisfying Eating on a Budget at http://newharbinger.com/56456.

MARGINALIZED IDENTITIES AND MINORITY STRESS

While anyone can experience an eating disorder, if you hold marginalized identities—that is, an identity that is outside the dominant group or one that experiences discrimination from the culture at large—you may be at increased risk (Barakat et al. 2023; Santoniccolo and Rollè 2024). Examples of marginalized identities include those who may be excluded or treated poorly due to race, gender identity, sexual orientation, body size, language, physical abilities, or age. Marginalized people are at increased risk of being unfairly treated due to biased beliefs and harmful practices of the most powerful and dominant group. Although BIPOC individuals are affected by eating disorders at similar rates as their white peers, they are about half as likely to be formally diagnosed with an eating disorder (Sonneville and Lipson 2018) and receive proper treatment.

Understandably, these experiences of stigma and discrimination in the social environment can cause mental and physical stress in the people who experience them. The chronic elevated stress associated with feeling "othered" increases the risk of negative physical and mental health outcomes. For example, people who experience higher levels of perceived weight stigma report higher levels of stress. This elevated stress alone places people at greater risk of type 2 diabetes and heart disease (Vadiveloo and Mattei 2017).

It's important to realize that having marginalized identities does not automatically mean that someone will suffer negative health consequences. In fact, having a marginalized identity may also lead to stronger ties with one's community, which can serve as a protective factor against stress and eating disorder development. For many, community and group connections offer a powerful healing environment from stigma and minority stress (Mueller et al. 2021).

TRAUMA

Many people describe a personal history of trauma in addition to the oppression described above. Research suggests that exposure to a traumatic experience is common in people with eating disorders (Trottier and MacDonald 2017). This can include any type of trauma, such as physical abuse, sexual abuse, emotional abuse, physical assault, sexual assault, living through an accident or natural disaster, combat trauma, experiencing the traumatic loss of someone close to you, experiencing a life-threatening illness or injury, or collective trauma (e.g., a global pandemic like COVID). It can also include medical trauma, systemic violence, and identity-based trauma such as anti-fat treatment, transphobia, and racialized scrutiny of physical appearance. If you have experienced trauma, it may be beneficial to find a therapist with experience treating trauma and eating disorders.

Have you experienced any of the above (food insecurity, marginalization, minority stress, and/or trauma)? If so, how has it impacted your relationship with eating and your body?

_____

_____

_____

_____

_____

_____

NEURODIVERSITY AND EATING DISORDERS

Neurodiversity is defined as differences in how people's brains function, particularly in communication, learning, sensory experiences, attention, and concentration. People with neurodivergence include those diagnosed with autism, attention deficit/hyperactivity disorder (ADHD), dyslexia (difficulties reading), and dyscalculia (difficulties learning and understanding numbers/math).

Research shows high rates of neurodivergence among people with eating disorders (Schröder et al. 2022; Yao et al. 2019). Traditional eating disorder interventions may require modifications for neurodiversity (Cobbaert and Rose 2023). We have tried to specify suggested modifications throughout CBT-WI.

Impacts of Eating Disorders

As stated by Christy Harrison, eating disorder dietitian and podcast host, eating disorders are "life thieves": They rob you of your mental and physical health, time, money, and overall well-being. Many people can relate to the statement that eating disorders take up a lot of "mental real estate" in their brains, leaving less time and energy for other aspects of life. You likely are already aware of how eating disorders have impacted your life, or you would not be here. This section aims to help you identify other ways your eating and body issues may affect you.

Physical Impacts

Numerous physical concerns can develop because of eating disorder symptoms. As noted earlier in the chapter, these medical issues can develop for people regardless of body size. Below are some common physical symptoms. Check off ones you have experienced and add any others not on the list.

- ☐ Heart problems—slow or fast heart rate, blood pressure changes, chest pain
- ☐ Shortness of breath
- ☐ Gastrointestinal problems—early fullness, constipation, nausea, involuntary vomiting, diarrhea, abdominal pain, heartburn/acid reflux, difficulty swallowing
- ☐ Bone weakness—low bone mineral density or stress fractures
- ☐ Muscle weakness
- ☐ Lightheadedness, dizziness, or fainting
- ☐ Low testosterone or estrogen or irregular menses
- ☐ Refeeding syndrome—a potentially fatal shifting of electrolytes
- ☐ Hypoglycemia/hyperglycemia
- ☐ Hair loss, dry or thinning hair, or lanugo (light, soft hair appearing on the face or body)
- ☐ Dry skin
- ☐ Brittle or discolored nails
- ☐ Feeling tired or fatigued
- ☐ Dental problems
- ☐ Feeling cold frequently
- ☐ Difficulties sleeping
- ☐ Decreased interest in sex or decreased arousal
- ☐ Changes in cholesterol levels
- ☐ Problems with fertility
- ☐ Anemia or vitamin deficiencies

☐ _____

☐ _____

☐ _____

It's important to note that some people with eating disorders may still have normal lab tests. However, that does not mean your eating concern is not serious. For this reason, we strongly encourage you to see a medical provider if you have had any of the physical symptoms noted above. Sleep issues are also very common for those with disordered eating, and we have included an online resource, Sleep and Disordered Eating, with information about these overlapping concerns at http://www.newharbinger.com/56456.

Emotional Impacts

Disordered eating can cause emotional changes, including anxiety and depression (Keys 1950). Below are common emotional symptoms. Check off ones you have experienced and add any others.

☐ Feeling down or depressed

☐ Feelings of guilt or shame

☐ Hopelessness about the future

☐ Thoughts of not wanting to be around or being better off dead

☐ Feeling unworthy

☐ Self-consciousness

☐ Irritability

☐ Anxiety

☐ _____

☐ _____

☐ _____

Suicide and Self-Harm

Thinking about eating and body image concerns can bring up many painful thoughts and emotions, including thoughts about self-harm. If you currently or previously had these thoughts, you are not alone. Having thoughts about suicide or self-harm doesn't mean that you will engage in these behaviors, but it's a good idea to seek support when this happens. It can be hard to ask for help if you're having thoughts of self-harm or suicide. Speaking about your thoughts with supportive people in your life may help increase support during difficult times.

If immediate social support isn't available—or you don't feel comfortable sharing with the people in your life—please reach out for help through the resources listed below. We understand it can be challenging to share these experiences and ask for help. Please know that your life matters, and you deserve help and support.

- Suicide and Crisis Lifeline: 988
- Crisis Text Line: Text HOME to 741741
- Trans Lifeline USA: (877) 565-8860
- Blackline: (800) 604-5841
- Don't Call the Police: https://dontcallthepolice.com
- Black Emotional and Mental Health Collective: https://beam.community/get-help-now
- Virtual Hope Box (free app available on IOS and Android)

Social or Occupational Impacts

People who struggle with eating often find that it impacts them socially or in terms of their school or work. It can be hard to focus on other activities when you are preoccupied with thoughts of food or your body. Check off any symptoms you have experienced below and add any others not listed.

- ☐ Conflicts with others
- ☐ Denying that your eating or low body weight is a problem (this is a state of mind known as *anosognosia*; the outside perspective your friends and family bring can be crucial in helping you get care)
- ☐ Difficulty connecting to others or feelings of isolation

☐   Difficulty concentrating on work or school

☐   Your eating or body-focused behaviors taking precedence over social, academic, or work activities

☐   Reduced involvement in hobbies and interests

☐   Difficulty being "spontaneous," sticking rigidly to your routines

☐   Concentration difficulties, inattention

☐   Lack of flexibility with your thinking

☐   Difficulty making decisions

☐   Obsessive preoccupation with food

☐   _____

☐   _____

☐   _____

☐   _____

☐   _____

☐   _____

Common Concerns About Change

You may notice concerns as you contemplate how your eating concerns have impacted you and what changes you want to make. This section will help address common worries.

I Have Noticed Physical Symptoms Related to My Eating Concerns, But What If I Don't Feel Comfortable with My Doctor?

Many people with eating behavior concerns have had negative interactions with health care providers when trying to seek help. It is best to identify health care providers who are weight-inclusive, when possible. One place to start is with our online resources at http://newharbinger.com/56456.

What If My Medical Provider Tells Me to Lose Weight?

Conflicting feedback from different members of your health care team can present challenges for people with eating disorder symptoms. It is important to understand that not all health care providers are familiar with eating disorders and the recommended treatments for these issues (Ayton and Ibrahim 2018). Many have had training that emphasized weight and may be unaware of how this focus can harm people with eating disorders.

If a provider recommends weight loss, consider the following steps:

1. Let them know you are experiencing symptoms of an eating disorder and are taking steps to recover.

2. Explain that part of healing from your eating disorder is reducing the focus on weight and shape.

3. Ask if it would be possible to avoid or minimize discussions about weight and food during appointments, and instead focus on the reason for your visit.

4. Ask if it would be possible to decline being weighed at the beginning of your appointments.

5. If you are working with a therapist or dietitian, they can provide support by collaborating with your medical providers to explain why weighing or recommending weight loss is harmful.

6. Consider bringing a Please Don't Weigh Me Card to your appointments; this can be found at http://newharbinger.com/56456.

I Want to Get Better, But Will I Gain Weight?

Fear of gaining weight or other body changes may be weighing on you (pun intended!). Maybe you have a strong desire to lose weight with the hope that it will improve your physical health. You may even be tempted to delay or avoid moving forward with recovery. If you find yourself worrying about weight gain and experience an urge to put this book aside, bear with us and know that you're not alone. If you are hoping to improve your health, many strategies in this book may help you. If you're looking for more support in this area, we recommend Margit Berman's *A Workbook of Acceptance-Based Approaches for Weight Concerns* and provide more links to weight-inclusive health resources online at http://www.newharbinger.com/56456.

In chapter 2, we will discuss how body weight is determined and why weight gain may happen during eating disorder recovery—and may even make you feel better! We can't promise that your body won't change, but we can reassure you that regular nourishment and addressing your relationship with food and your body can help improve your health, well-being, and quality of life. This workbook will provide you with support to address anxiety and fear related to changes in weight.

Can I Get Better?

The good news is that many people with eating disorders can improve their symptoms and reduce the impact of their eating disorder on their quality of life. Research on CBT for eating disorders has shown that approximately two-thirds of people who complete it experience a significant improvement in symptoms (Fairburn et al. 2015). Most research on CBT for eating disorders has not included people in larger bodies or those with marginalized identities. That said, we believe the adaptations we suggest in this book will enable the treatment to be tailored for individuals with diverse identities.

Are You Ready to Make Changes?

Change can be challenging, and sometimes it can be helpful to consider how changing your eating behaviors may improve your quality of life. The following worksheet (also available online) will help you consider potential positive aspects and challenges of your current symptoms and assess your readiness to change.

Readiness to Change

How do the eating disorder behaviors you are trying to change negatively impact your life?

Examples:

I don't have a lot of energy when I restrict/diet.

I feel guilt and shame after binge eating.

I feel physically uncomfortable after overeating.

I'm stuck in a pattern of dieting/weight cycling.

I can't stop thinking about food.

I hide food or eat in secret.

_____

_____

_____

_____

_____

_____

_____

What are some of the ways these eating disorder behaviors are helping you?

Examples:

They help me cope with difficult emotions.

It's easier to fit in with diet culture around me.

They help me control my weight.

I'm engaging in some of my eating behaviors with friends/family.

I enjoy the foods I am eating and worry about feeling deprived if I make changes.

_____

_____

_____

_____

_____

_____

_____

_____

What challenges may arise as you make changes?

Examples:

It will take a lot of time to complete the workbook and make changes to my routines.

I may have to find other ways to manage emotions.

I am scared about gaining weight.

_____

_____

_____

_____

_____

_____

_____

_____

If you decide to make changes, what are some positive changes you hope for?

Examples:

I want to feel less restricted about food choices.

I would like to improve my relationship with food.

I want to improve my body image.

I am hoping to feel better physically.

I want to have more energy.

_____

_____

_____

_____

_____

_____

_____

_____

Thinking about all the positive aspects and challenges of making changes to your eating behaviors, how ready are you feeling to change at this time? Circle a number below to rate your current readiness:

1	2	3	4	5	6	7	8	9	10

Not at all ready
to change

Completely ready
to change

List your top three to five reasons for change.

1. _____

2. _____

3. _____

4. _____

5. _____

Some people find it helpful to keep this list available to review. You can either return to this page in the workbook, take a picture to save on your phone, or consider writing these reasons on a small index card to keep with you. Reviewing why you want to change your eating behaviors can be helpful when things feel challenging.

Others find it helpful to take the time to imagine what their life will be like in the future once their symptoms improve. Take a moment to describe what your recovered life looks like. How will your day-to-day life, relationships, and experiences with your body, food, and eating change?

_____

_____

_____

_____

_____

_____

Summary of Takeaways

Congratulations on finishing chapter 1! Here are some takeaways:

- Eating disorders do not have a "look": They affect people of all genders, ages, races, ethnicities, body shapes, weights, sexual orientations, and socioeconomic statuses.

- If your identity has not traditionally been represented as somebody who is at risk of developing an eating disorder (i.e., thin white cisgender women), you may be less likely to identify with having one. Even though your symptoms may have been overlooked, you deserve to get treatment!

- Disordered eating can significantly impact your physical, mental, and social health.

- We don't know exactly what causes eating disorders. However, you may be at elevated risk due to dieting and factors outside of your control—like genetics, discrimination, oppression, trauma, limited access to food, and societal appearance ideals.

- We don't need to know what caused your eating problems to help you get better. CBT-WI offers strategies that can help all people with eating issues.

Reflection

What are your takeaways from chapter 1? Take a moment to reflect on anything that surprised you or aspects of the chapter that felt relevant to you. If you are currently working with a therapist, consider sharing these observations with them.

_____

_____

_____

_____

_____

When to Move on to Chapter 2

- You've identified resources needed to keep yourself safe, if needed (such as finding a medical provider or adding a crisis text number to your phone).

- You've completed the Readiness to Change worksheet.

Chapter 2

Understanding Your Eating Behaviors

In chapter 1, you learned about how eating disorders develop. In this chapter, we explore factors that maintain disordered eating. One of the common concerns people report is "loss of control" over eating. You may call this binge eating, "emotional eating," or "food addiction." We will help you see that it's usually food restriction—or a mindset that food *should* be restricted—that needs to be addressed. Unfortunately, our culture has vilified binge eating and praised food restriction.

Factors That Maintain Disordered Eating

Binge eating rarely persists without restriction. Food restriction, weight concerns, the idea of "managing" one's weight, and weight suppression are four factors that often maintain an individual's disordered eating after it has started. After exploring these factors, you will create your symptom map to understand what keeps your eating disorder going.

Food Restriction

Although many people associate food restriction with anorexia nervosa, it is a component of most eating disorders. Restriction can also be more than just limiting your food intake. It can be related to unspoken rules from family, peers, medical providers, or the media about what you should eat. It can also include the intent to restrict, which can change eating behaviors (Hart and Chiovari

1998). For example, someone may think, "I've been eating so badly this weekend, I need to get back on my diet on Monday." Even if food intake is not actually restricted, these thoughts can trigger behaviors such as binge eating, eating in secret, or purging. As you start to understand your thoughts and feelings about eating, you may find that you have been engaging in more restriction than you realized. The following are some other common types of restrictions.

Check off the types of restriction that you have experienced and add any others not listed.

☐ Limiting portions/calories

☐ Limiting types of food or food groups

☐ Limiting times of day you can eat

☐ Delaying eating even when you are hungry

☐ Only allowing yourself to eat after physical activity

☐ Not eating or limiting eating when you are with others

☐ Not eating in certain situations (e.g., at restaurants, at work)

☐ Thinking about or spending time researching diets

☐ Not eating all day to "save up" for a big or celebratory meal

☐ _____

☐ _____

☐ _____

Weight Concerns

Weight is a complex topic. There are many misconceptions about the ability to control body weight and the connection between weight and health. Unfortunately, weight science is often misunderstood by health care providers. While a full critique of the often-misunderstood relationship between weight and health is beyond the scope of this workbook, we provide resources online at http://www.newharbinger.com/56456 to explore the limitations of focusing solely on weight loss as a path to better health.

You are likely familiar with the BMI. Recently, the American Medical Association (AMA) recommended against the use of the BMI due to its historical harm, use for racist exclusion, and basis in data collected from nonrepresentative groups (Jakubek 2023; Flegal 2023). Further, overreliance on BMI leads to delays in eating disorder treatment for people in larger bodies (Ramaswamy and Ramaswamy 2023).

The BMI was inspired by insurance actuarial tables created in the 1800s by Adolphe Quetelet, a Belgian mathematician—not a physician—searching for the "average" man. Deemed "ideal weight tables," they produced a formula to identify any "outliers" who could be charged more for life insurance. The tables were never intended to be a health measurement. The BMI was not used for health purposes until 1972 when Ancel Keys formally coined the term "BMI" based roughly on Quetelet's formulas (Strings 2019).

As highlighted by Aubrey Gordon in her 2020 book, *What We Don't Talk About When We Talk About Fat*, and Sabrina Strings's 2019 book, *Fearing the Black Body: The Racial Origins of Fat Phobia*, the BMI was based only on white European men, ignoring women and people of color. Research shows Black people often have higher BMIs because of higher bone density and muscle mass, but lower death rates at the same BMI. This demonstrates an example of the racial bias inherent in the BMI. For more, see Da'Shaun Harrison's 2021 book, *Belly of the Beast*, and other resources provided online at http://www.newharbinger.com/56456.

Due to these and other limitations, we recommend against computing your BMI. It does not provide valuable information about your health or the severity of your eating disorder.

How Much Can You Really "Manage" Your Body Weight?

Our society and its medical system maintain a strong focus on "managing" one's weight to promote positive health outcomes. Whether it's medications for weight loss, crash diets, or even a "lifestyle change" program prescribed by a medical doctor, it's hard to go longer than a few hours without seeing some kind of advertisement for weight control products. As a result, it is widely believed that people have control over their weight. In truth, your weight is similar to other vital signs, such as heart rate and blood pressure. There may be certain things you can do to lower your heart rate in the short term—such as taking some deep breaths or lying down—but ultimately, many other factors are at play. Genetics, age, overall stress level, medical conditions—or for those who menstruate, time in your menstrual cycle—all influence your resting heart rate.

Similarly, numerous factors influence our weight at any given time. Fluid and food intake, clothing, time of day, medications, hormonal changes, bladder storage, bowel movements, and the scale used all contribute to weight fluctuations. It is also important to note that body weight fluctuations are common. Therefore, we cannot determine weight based on a single data point; trends over weeks, months, and years provide more accurate data.

Many people are either unaware or unwilling to accept that our weight is also predetermined mainly by genetics and biological factors outside our control. Coined by a physician and nutrition researcher in the 1980s, the *set point theory* (Bennett 1983) directly contradicts the idea that body weight can be "managed" in the long term. This theory suggests instead that each body has a biologically preset weight range that it is destined to maintain. Powerful unmodifiable factors and bodily processes—such as genetics, aging, menopause, childbirth, diseases, and continued attempts to lose weight by dieting and restriction—impact a person's set point weight. Fighting your set point by engaging in restriction is not sustainable and often leads to other disordered eating behaviors.

Before reading this book, what were you taught about your body weight and ability to control it? What messages did you get about your need to control your weight? Where did these messages come from?

_____

_____

_____

_____

Weight Suppression

Human bodies exist in a variety of shapes and sizes. When a person of any size tries to reduce their size to one smaller than that intended by their genetics, binge eating may be the body's natural defense to avoid death by starvation and return the body to a higher weight that better supports its needs.

Weight loss decreases the body's metabolism and the amount of energy it burns, while also increasing appetite. The hormone leptin, which sends satiety signals to the brain, is believed to play a role in this process. Studies indicate that people with high weight suppression—that is, who have lost a lot of weight—appear to have lower levels of leptin (Keel et al. 2017).

Weight suppression occurs when your body is at a weight lower than its natural set point, which is the body's favored weight. You will experience symptoms of starvation when you keep your body below its set point. Weight suppression is like holding a beach ball underwater. You can keep it below the surface with much effort, but as soon as you relax, it pops back up. It takes considerable effort to override your body's natural needs, and eventually, your body will push back to reclaim balance. Weight suppression is dangerous for people in all body sizes and maintains eating disorder symptoms.

Knowing whether you are weight-suppressed can give important information about whether you need to gain weight to recover from your eating issues. Note that this can be true even if you are in a bigger body and have been told by others that you should lose weight. It's okay to skip this worksheet (also available online) if you don't want to focus on your weight now. You may want to come back to this later.

Are You Weight Suppressed?

Think about your current weight or body size. You don't need to weigh yourself for this activity.

What was your highest weight as an adult?

_____

If your current weight is lower than your highest adult weight, you could be weight suppressed. Does that fit with your experience? Have you been at a higher weight than you are currently? What might that mean?

_____

_____

_____

Think about your body size during childhood. Was your body average, small, or big? What were your memories of your body size?

_____

_____

_____

How would you describe your body size now? If you find it helpful, we have a link to a resource that describes body sizes at http://newharbinger.com/56456.

_____

_____

_____

If you considered yourself bigger as a child, and smaller on the size spectrum now, you could be weight suppressed. Consider that your childhood body knew what to do. Your body was growing along a certain size trajectory. What might have happened to change that?

_____

_____

_____

Do you have genetic family members who are in bigger bodies? Or who are making great efforts to suppress their weight? What might that say about your genetics?

_____

_____

Consider that maybe you are destined to have a bigger body than many of your genetic family members. What feelings does that bring up?

_____

_____

Are you the same weight as you were in high school? Or striving for that weight? Bodies are supposed to change over time. Although diet culture may lead us to believe otherwise, you aren't meant to fit into your high school jeans for life!

_____

Do you gain weight easily, such as after a vacation? This could be another sign of weight suppression. When has this happened?

_____

_____

After reflecting on the questions above, do you believe your body might be weight suppressed? Why or why not?

_____

_____

We know that this can be scary to think about, but consider the cost of fighting your body's set point. It is likely maintaining your disordered eating. Remember the symptoms we discussed in chapter 1? Many of these are costs of weight suppression and can improve significantly with proper nourishment and weight restoration. Please also check out our handout, Impacts of Undereating and Weight Suppression, at http://newharbinger.com/56456.

Our colleague Rachel Millner wrote, "One of the most unexpected things in my life is that fatness has had more of an impact on my liberation than almost anything else. I thought it would be thinness that set me free, but when I was thin in the midst of an eating disorder, I was never more trapped. It was only when I got fat while healing that I was truly set free." She also provided the following prompt, which we invite you to reflect on here.

What would it be like to open yourself up to the possibility that this could be true for you? Will getting/staying fat liberate you? What if freedom is not found in thinness as you've been told, but in letting your body grow?

_____

_____

_____

_____

We will provide you with more support on this topic as you continue through the workbook. We recognize that body liberation may be more or less accessible depending on other identities you hold or access to other advantages in life. For example, a white person may not experience discrimination based on their skin color and may have an easier time fitting in, even when fat.

Symptom Mapping

Some people find it helpful to create a visual representation of how their eating disorder developed and is maintained. The map below (adapted from Fairburn 2008) provides an example, and we will help you create your own.

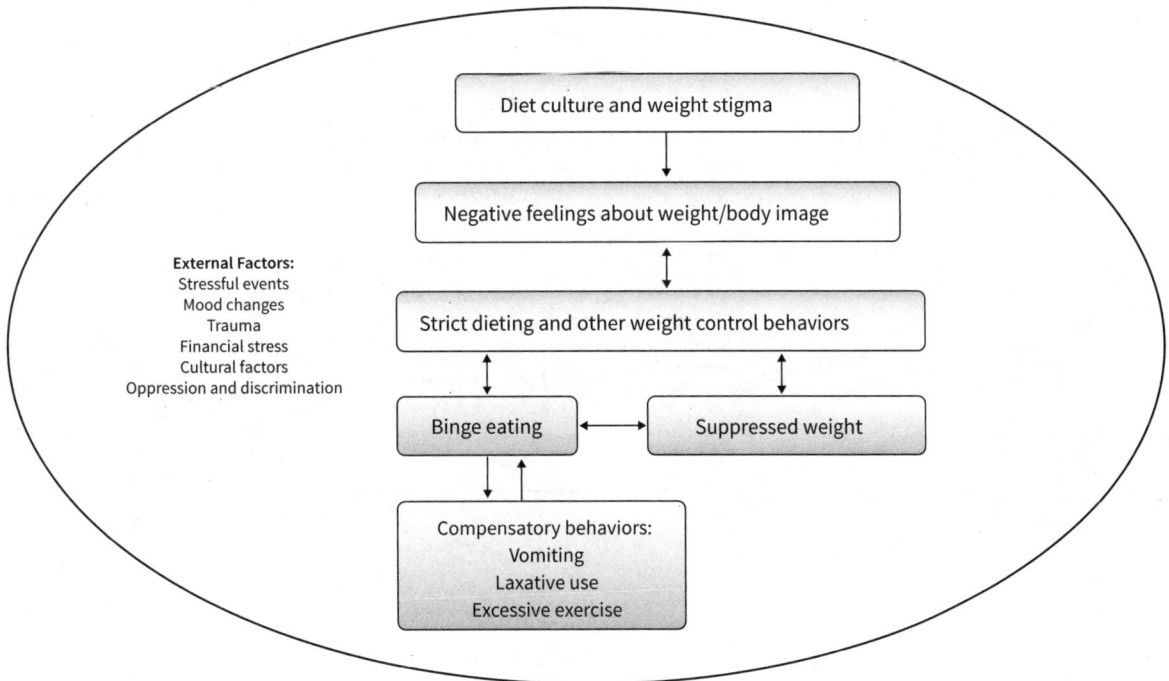

External Factors:
Stressful events
Mood changes
Trauma
Financial stress
Cultural factors
Oppression and discrimination

Diet culture and weight stigma

Negative feelings about weight/body image

Strict dieting and other weight control behaviors

Binge eating

Suppressed weight

Compensatory behaviors:
Vomiting
Laxative use
Excessive exercise

On the following pages, you can see examples of symptom maps from other people who have struggled with their eating and body image.

Jamal's Symptom Map

Jamal, a fifty-year-old bisexual man, has been coping with his eating disorder for years. He feels frustrated by his inability to control his eating. His friends at the gym have been following a ketogenic diet to "bulk," and so he's followed suit. In addition to his eating and shape concerns, he feels frustrated by the lack of acceptance by his siblings now that he's recently come out as bisexual and started dating his boyfriend.

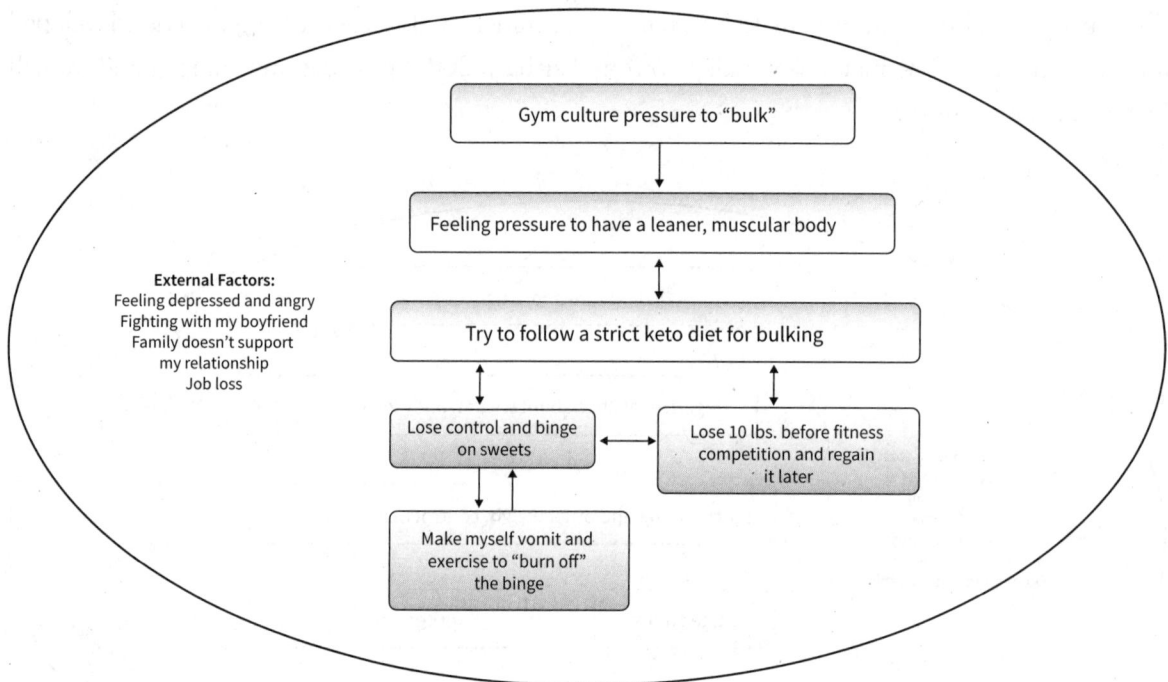

External Factors:
Feeling depressed and angry
Fighting with my boyfriend
Family doesn't support
my relationship
Job loss

Gym culture pressure to "bulk"

Feeling pressure to have a leaner, muscular body

Try to follow a strict keto diet for bulking

Lose control and binge on sweets

Lose 10 lbs. before fitness competition and regain it later

Make myself vomit and exercise to "burn off" the binge

Crystal's Symptom Map

Crystal has been dieting for about five years. The daughter of immigrants, she gained weight in high school and was teased by her peers for being fat. With encouragement from her parents, who were also concerned about her fitting in, she started attending a weight loss program when she was twenty. She lost weight and began to have an easier time finding clothes that fit. She meticulously maintains this weight by limiting her intake to coffee for breakfast, salad for lunch, and a small dinner. She eats all her meals at home and resists going out with friends because she believes she will overeat. She thinks about food frequently when she is bored at work. Recently, she noticed that her energy level is low and her hair is falling out.

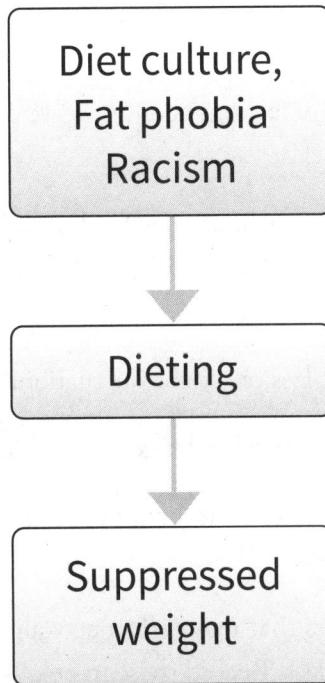

Can you identify with the maps we included? If not, how would it look different for you?

_____

_____

Creating your symptom map can be a helpful step toward understanding your disordered eating. The following worksheet (also available online) will help you create your own map. Over the course of the workbook, you can add to this map—it's okay if you aren't yet sure what this fully looks like! It's also okay if your map looks nothing like the ones above.

Your Personal Symptom Map

To create your eating behavior symptom map, respond to the following reflection questions. Then, use the blank space to compose your map. You may not have entries in every box.

1. What were some of your experiences with diet culture, weight stigma, or discrimination? Describe these in box 1.

2. Have you experienced negative feelings about your weight or body image? Record these in box 2.

3. Have you attempted to restrict or limit your food intake in response to boxes 1 and 2? Have you experienced food insecurity or difficulty planning or organizing meals? If so, describe in box 3.

4. Have you experienced weight loss or weight fluctuation? Describe this in box 4.

5. Have you experienced loss of control or binge eating? Describe this in box 5.

6. Do you use any behaviors to try to cancel out or "undo" what you've eaten? Record this in box 6.

7. List additional external factors that may influence your eating. Examples could include stressful events or mood changes. Record these in box 7.

My Personal
Symptom Map

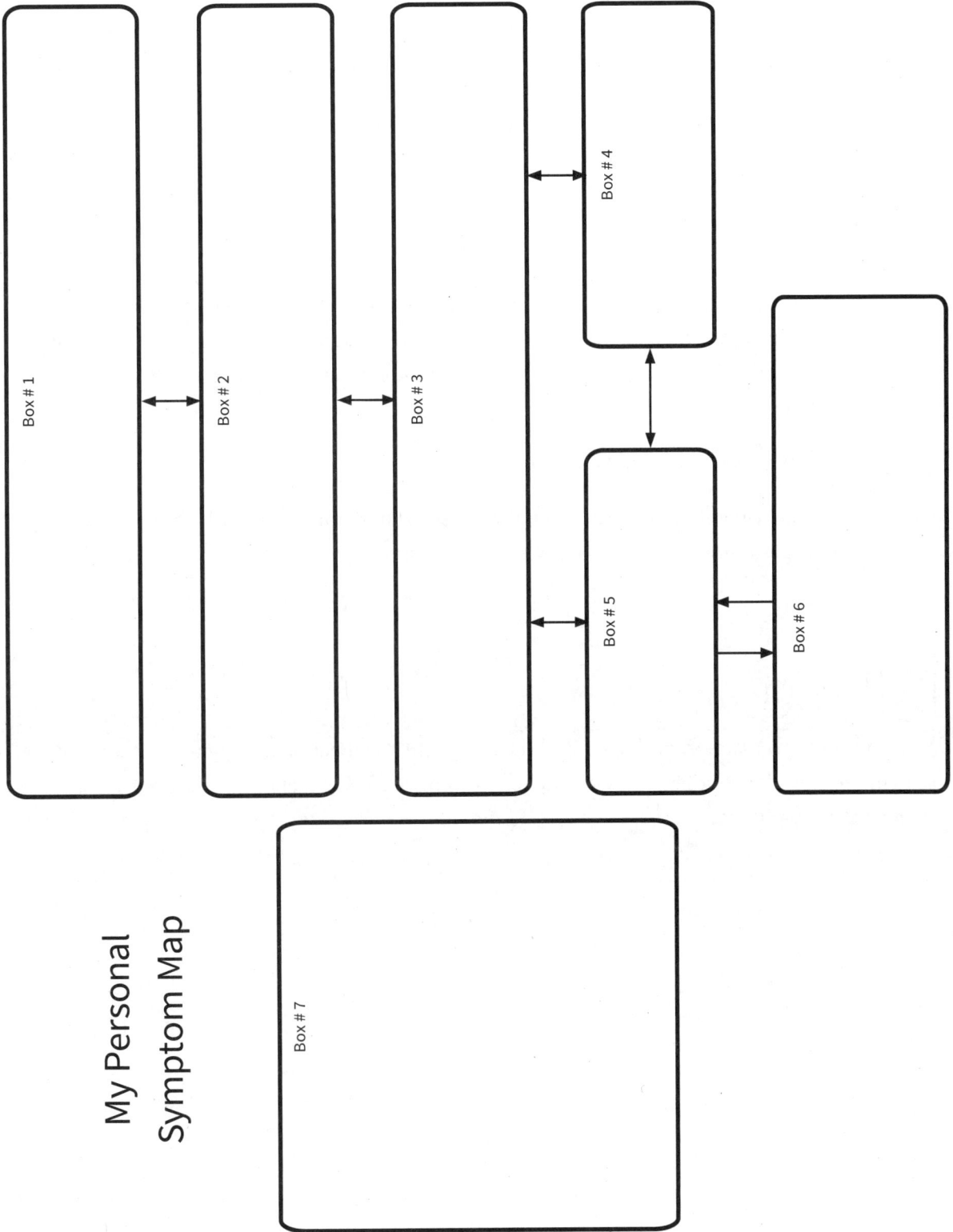

Box # 1

Box # 2

Box # 3

Box # 4

Box # 5

Box # 6

Box # 7

Summary of Takeaways

Another chapter down—way to go! Here are some takeaways from chapter 2.

- Although food restriction is most often associated with anorexia, it plays a role in driving all eating disorders.

- The BMI is an outdated, flawed, and biased measure. It is not a measure of health or self-worth.

- There is only so much that you can do to control your weight. Similar to other metrics like our heart rate, we can do things in the short term to make it go up and down, but at the end of the day, factors outside of our control—such as genetics and medical conditions—determine it.

- People in all body sizes can be weight suppressed.

- Symptom mapping is a powerful way to understand how our society influences behaviors that keep you stuck in a cycle of disordered eating.

Reflection

What are your takeaways from chapter 2? Take a moment to reflect on anything that surprised you or aspects of the chapter that felt especially relevant to you. What feelings or thoughts came up as you read the information?

_____

_____

_____

_____

_____

When to Move on to Chapter 3

- You've completed My Personal Symptom Map.

Chapter 3

Self-Monitoring

In this chapter, you will learn about self-monitoring and its importance. As you progress through this workbook, we invite you to record your eating behaviors, internal experiences (such as thoughts or emotions), and the situations in which they occur. This is called "self-monitoring," and it can help you investigate your behaviors like a detective. Some say this process helps them distance themselves from their eating concerns and become aware of other factors that may impact their behaviors.

Self-monitoring is optional, flexible, and should not cause harm. We will provide our rationale for using these strategies, and you can decide whether they are right for you. Remember that you won't have to self-monitor forever, but we find this an illuminating activity in the initial part of the process. We will guide you on when and how to stop self-monitoring as you progress.

Reasons to Self-Monitor

Self-monitoring is a cornerstone of CBT because it provides critical information about your symptoms and how to intervene. In CBT for eating disorders, recording eating and other related behaviors is an opportunity to learn more about why you do what you do. Self-monitoring serves four main purposes:

1. It provides important information about your eating behaviors and emotional experiences. Most people have difficulty remembering what they thought or felt yesterday or even a few hours ago. Self-monitoring can help you become aware of how thoughts,

sensations, and situations contribute to your disordered eating. For example, you might identify that you are going too long without eating or not eating enough. You might also identify emotional or situational triggers for certain behaviors. Alternatively, you might identify situations and factors that help prevent disordered eating episodes.

2. It highlights changes you can make that may help you recover. Real-time recording will alert you to decision points where you can change patterns you thought were outside your control. It provides quick feedback as you try different strategies.

3. It will create an ongoing log of your progress—you can look back at previous self-monitoring notes and see how far you've come.

4. Finally, self-monitoring allows you to take more time to reflect on your current needs. This awareness can help you adopt a different behavior or coping strategy to better serve you.

Instructions for Self-Monitoring

We invite you to write down eating behaviors, emotions, thoughts, and relevant events as soon as they happen. This "real-time" self-monitoring will help ensure you don't forget important details of your experience.

How you record information is not important—the format that is most convenient for you is fine. In this book, we provide a self-monitoring form (also available online) so you can begin recording your experiences today. We also include an example of a completed form—we hope this sparks ideas about the types of experiences you might choose to write down.

If the form doesn't work for you, that's okay! You might use a recovery-focused app such as Recovery Record or Brighter Bite, or a notebook, journal, or Google document. Avoid calorie-counting weight loss apps, which can focus more on restrictive and dieting behaviors. You might find recording on your phone via an app or creating a memo or document is most convenient. Some people also take photos of their meals and put them into a document later. The important thing is to keep a record of the context every time you eat or engage in disordered eating behavior.

What to Record

You should record the following details:

- The date and time—this will help you keep track of changes as you progress.

- The type of food you consume. Just estimate the quantities—don't worry about precision. Don't weigh or measure the food, record calories, or record macronutrients. Instead, describe it generally: one chicken breast, a handful of peanuts, one protein bar, a medium-size bowl of cereal, two scoops of ice cream, or a turkey and cheese sandwich with mayo.

- Group all foods consumed in each eating episode and include liquids.

- Your location when you were eating. Include details—if you were at home, were you sitting at the table or on the couch? Where were you, and who was with you if you were out?

- Relevant situations, thoughts, or feelings. Note whether you had an argument or intense emotion before eating that may have influenced your behavior. Even if you are unsure that it had an impact, it's good to put down more information—these may be dots you can connect later.

- Related behaviors—including "binges"; elimination through vomiting, laxatives, or other diet aids—and the time at which they occurred. Any of these behaviors should be recorded, even if they didn't occur during an eating episode. If no food was consumed at the time, just leave the food section blank.

- Any movement, whether for weight control, athletic training, leisure, or significant walking or standing. Note the time, amount, and type of movement you engaged in. It is also important to document your feelings before, during, and after this activity.

Self-Monitoring Form Example

Date: Saturday, July 10

Time	Type Meal (M) Snack (S) Other (O)	Food Intake	Location	Behaviors Restrict (R) Binge (B) Purge (P) Laxative (L)	Thoughts/Feelings/Situation
11 a.m.	M	2 slices of toast with Nutella, 2 scrambled eggs, vanilla latte with whole milk	Alone in my kitchen		Worried about what to have for dinner tonight
2 p.m.	S	1 mini orange and 1 string cheese		R	Didn't want to eat, but knew that I should. Frustrated because person I was hoping to hear from wasn't texting me back
3 p.m.	S	Vanilla latte with low-fat milk		R	I'm hungry now, but trying to wait for dinner
6 p.m.	M	Bowl of chips with multiple spoonfuls of guacamole, chicken quesadilla, rice and beans, margarita			Feeling self-conscious; couldn't stop eating the chips
10 p.m.	S?	2 pints of ice cream, 2 sleeves of cookies		B/P	Very upset and angry with myself; can't stop thinking about interactions at dinner; binge eating and purging was a distraction

Movement:

9 a.m.: 90-minute workout video for weight loss and to be able to eat today; felt tired

4 p.m.: 45-minute walk with friend to increase steps; felt I didn't get my heart rate up enough

Self-Monitoring Form

Date:					
Time	**Type** Meal (M) Snack (S) Other (O)	**Food Intake**	**Location**	**Behaviors** Restrict (R) Binge (B) Purge (P) Laxative (L)	**Thoughts/Feelings/ Situation**

Movement:

Now that you understand why self-monitoring is beneficial and what a completed record looks like, consider whether this strategy could be helpful to you. Remember, this is optional, and we recommend holding off on it if it seems like it may cause you harm. We will also include some tips below for making the process simpler and more manageable if the example above seems overwhelming.

Common Concerns About Self-Monitoring

Many people feel reluctant to self-monitor. It's normal to worry or feel self-conscious about your eating habits. You may be tempted to leave out information or avoid recording to reduce feelings of guilt or shame. For some people, the self-disclosure of writing it all down can feel scary because it makes the behaviors "real" and more difficult to avoid. We live by the motto "Name it to tame it," which means that the act alone of writing or "naming" your internal experiences in the thoughts and feelings column of your record can, in and of itself, help you learn about your needs and feel more at ease.

We also want to acknowledge that some people may have previously participated in weight loss treatment where other health care providers criticized their eating and food choices. Some food records and apps recommended for self-monitoring focus on calories and macronutrients. These apps can increase disordered eating (Levinson, Fewell, and Brosof 2017; Linardon and Messer 2019). Let us reassure you that our process will be different. CBT-WI self-monitoring will not criticize or shame you for breaking a diet rule, going off your diet, eating certain foods, or eating "too much." This type of self-monitoring will not ask you to count calories. The situations in which you don't eat enough are the ones that most concern us. You do not need to share your completed forms with anyone, although as you become more comfortable with the process, you may want to share them with your treatment providers, who can provide support and feedback.

- *Jessica's Story*

   Jessica is a divorced woman in her thirties who recently decided to seek out treatment to help with her night eating. She tried raising these concerns with her doctor in the past, and they encouraged her to limit eating after 7 p.m. and try using a calorie-tracking app to lose weight. Jessica found that the app caused her anxiety about eating to skyrocket. She found herself trying to stay within the recommended calorie limit during the day and then felt too ashamed to log the food she was eating at night after her evening meal.

   When her new therapist recommended self-monitoring to help with her nighttime eating, she was reluctant and concerned that the same cycle would start all over again. Her therapist assured her that she would not need to count calories, track her weight, or anything similar with this self-monitoring. Instead, she could briefly describe the timing and location of her meals and snacks, along with any thoughts, feelings, or other reactions she noted around these times. Her therapist also assured Jessica that the purpose of the self-monitoring was not to punish herself or feel worse about her eating. Instead, she could use the results to observe patterns in her eating that could help her make small changes moving forward. She did not even need to share her self-monitoring with her therapist during the first few weeks if that helped her feel more comfortable.

Jessica felt relieved and was able to start self-monitoring for a few days at a time. Within a few weeks, she realized that she was still eating insufficiently during the day, which increased her hunger at night. Jessica also noticed that her depression and boredom seemed to worsen at times, and she was able to speak with her therapist about other coping strategies. She worked on eating flexibly in the evening and incorporated an evening snack. Jessica eventually decreased the frequency of her self-monitoring, but she knew it could be a useful tool if she ever needed it again in the future.

Like Jessica, many people worry that self-monitoring will increase both their preoccupation and their distress about food and eating. In the short term, this could happen. However, this usually only lasts for a week or so. The benefits of the essential information your records provide far outweigh these initial costs. Sometimes things are harder before they become easier. Recording your eating and behaviors—even those you find most shameful—will help you greatly. Self-monitoring alerts you to the factors that contribute to these behaviors. And once you are aware of them, you can identify strategies to help change them.

Some people worry self-monitoring will be inconvenient or require too much effort. We encourage you not to overthink it—realistically, each eating occasion should only need about two minutes to record. Compare this to the time you spend on your phone daily. It's nothing! Recording in real time is quicker than waiting because you won't struggle to recall details. It will become almost automatic once you've turned this into a habit.

If you have recorded your eating habits before and found it unhelpful, we encourage you to try again. We have seen it provide people perspective on what they're doing, thinking, and feeling. Many people find that the monitoring methods described above are easier and less time-consuming than expected. If you are working with a therapist and/or dietitian, they can also help you find the right self-monitoring method.

If you initially find recording details about your eating too upsetting, consider completing the other columns on the self-monitoring form to help identify some of your current eating-related patterns. Remember, if self-monitoring leads you to feel too overwhelmed, overloaded, or triggered, it is okay to skip this step for now. We recommend you complete the Weekly Progress Tracker, which we will introduce in the next chapter.

Weight Monitoring

Unlike other CBT treatments, this workbook does not include weight monitoring. We believe that weighing yourself weekly may not be helpful unless you are weight suppressed and working with a provider to restore weight. If you are frequently weighing yourself, you may find it helpful to stop or reduce weighing to once a week. Chapter 7 will provide strategies to help you. Forced weighing may be harmful because it can hinder efforts to change behaviors, intensify fears about food, and make it more difficult for you to focus on recovery (Froreich, Ratcliffe, and Vartanian 2020). Additionally, this practice can increase concern about weight and reinforce weight stigma (McEntee, Philip, and Phelan 2023).

Depending on your situation, a medical professional may need to monitor your weight and vital signs (e.g., blood pressure, heart rate, and electrolyte levels) for your physical safety. If you are weight suppressed, weight restoration is essential. If you are uncertain about the role of weight in your recovery, we recommend finding an eating disorder provider who uses a Health at Every Size or weight-inclusive approach. It is a common misconception among medical and mental health providers that people in larger bodies cannot have a life-threatening eating disorder. Research shows that people can suffer from serious side effects regardless of their body size or weight (Golden and Mehler 2020). Refer to the online resources for assistance in locating a weight-inclusive provider and accessing weight-neutral health information.

> How does it feel to think about not weighing yourself during CBT-WI? Do you feel relief, anxiety, or something in between?
>
> _____
>
> _____
>
> _____
>
> _____

Summary of Takeaways

Congratulations on finishing chapter 3! Here are some takeaways from chapter 3.

- Self-monitoring helps you learn about your patterns to identify your needs.

- You can flexibly self-monitor in a way that meets your needs.

Reflection

What are your takeaways from chapter 3? How are you feeling about starting the self-monitoring process?

_____

_____

_____

When to Move on to Chapter 4

- You've tried self-monitoring for a week or decided to hold off.

- You've become more aware of your eating patterns.

Chapter 4

Regular Eating and Meal Planning

Welcome to chapter 4! Congratulations on completing self-monitoring. Even if you couldn't make it happen daily, these efforts add up. In this chapter, we review your self-monitoring and introduce regular eating and meal planning. Complete the following worksheet (also available online) to reflect on the process of self-monitoring.

Reflection on Self-Monitoring Process

After self-monitoring for one week, consider the reflection questions below.

How was the process of self-monitoring?

_____

_____

How did you choose to record? Are there any changes you want to make?

_____

_____

If you didn't self-monitor, what got in the way? How did you feel about it?

_____

_____

_____

_____

Did you forget to record? Were there times when you chose not to record certain behaviors?

_____

_____

_____

Were there columns that were difficult to complete? What do you think made it difficult?

_____

_____

_____

Troubleshooting Problems with Self-Monitoring

Below are common barriers to self-monitoring. If you struggled to self-monitor, see whether your reasons match what we identified and consider the strategies we've listed to address them. There is also a space for additional reasons you might have identified—we encourage you to identify a strategy to help you move forward.

Problem	Potential Strategy
I forgot.	Try setting reminders on your phone (apps offer an option to turn on reminders to self-monitor), putting the forms in a well-traveled place (e.g., where you usually eat), wearing a colored bracelet to try to remember, or using a sticky note to cue you.
I'm embarrassed.	Feeling embarrassed about your behaviors is common. Remember, you're not alone! Consider that this is an important step on the path toward change. What might you say to someone you care about who is experiencing something similar? Make a pros and cons list for completing self-monitoring (see below).
It made me more obsessive or anxious.	Sometimes, this happens. It usually gets better if you stick with it. Can you continue for one more week and see whether it gets easier? Or pause and come back to it? Would it be easier to keep photos of meals? A side note: Be sure to write down your eating habits *after* they occur, rather than preplanning and trying to stick to a plan—remember, this isn't another diet! This isn't forever, and it's to learn where you can *add* versus *take away*.
I don't believe it will help me.	We understand that you may have doubts. In our experience, it is extremely helpful. Remember that change doesn't happen overnight. We also give you full permission not to change your behaviors yet—you're only collecting information. Would you give it another try this week?
It's too inconvenient.	Can you try again using a different format? For example, if you tried to use paper forms, consider trying an app instead. If the app is cumbersome, try the notes on your phone or photos.
I left the Thoughts and Feelings column blank.	We see this a lot! It's not uncommon for people to struggle with identifying their thoughts and emotions. First, note the times that eating feels distressing or you experience urges to use disordered behaviors. If you're having trouble labeling your experiences, feel free to use the Feelings Wheel in the online resources at http://newharbinger.com/5645.
Other: _____	Potential strategy: _____

If you are on the fence, you might consider completing this pros and cons list.

Potential Pros of Self-Monitoring

_____

_____

_____

_____

_____

Potential Cons of Self-Monitoring

_____

_____

_____

_____

_____

If you decide that self-monitoring is not right for you now, you can still benefit from this workbook. If you feel more ready to engage in self-monitoring at any time in the workbook, return to this chapter for more guidance.

If you implemented self-monitoring this past week, please use the following worksheet (also available online) to review your logs. We will spend the following two chapters reviewing and reflecting on what you recorded.

Reflection on Self-Monitoring Content

What did you notice about your eating patterns?

_____

_____

_____

How long did you typically go between meals and snacks?

_____

_____

Were any meals or snacks skipped?

_____

_____

_____

Were there long gaps between meals (i.e., did you go longer than three or four hours without eating)?

_____

_____

_____

Was your eating schedule similar on most days, or did it vary?

_____

_____

_____

Did anything surprise you?

_____

_____

_____

How do you feel about your eating?

_____

_____

_____

Were there days during which you could eat more regularly than others? What did you notice about those days?

_____

_____

_____

Regular Eating

Now that you have a baseline of your eating patterns, we will help you gradually make changes to support recovery. Eating for recovery is built on the foundation of regular eating. It's important to eat adequate amounts of food consistently throughout each day, permitting yourself to choose broadly from the foods you can access.

We will focus first on what we mean by regular eating; later, we will address quantity and variety. Regular eating—the "guideline of threes," or 3-3-3 (3 meals, 3 snacks every 3–4 hours)—is perhaps the most important skill for recovery from disordered eating. Research has shown that people who engage in regular eating are more likely to reduce their eating disorder symptoms, specifically those who struggle with binge eating (Ellison et al. 2016; Sivyer et al. 2020). Regular eating is important for individuals with *all* types of eating disorders and for people in all sizes of bodies. It is also crucial for people with digestive issues and medical concerns such as diabetes. Neurodivergent people and those who use medication that affects appetite can also greatly benefit from regular eating. Regular eating is sometimes called "mechanical eating" because it is supposed to occur like clockwork with regularity and predictability, rather than relying on hunger cues alone, which can often be unreliable.

Basic Recommended Eating Schedule

Regular eating involves eating something roughly every three waking hours. This generally comprises three meals and two or three snacks a day. This might look something like:

- Breakfast (within an hour of waking)

- Morning snack (if breakfast and lunch are more than four hours apart)

- Lunch

- Afternoon snack (midway between lunch and dinner)

- Dinner

- Evening snack (especially if up longer than four hours after dinner)

- And if you stay up extra late, are weight suppressed, or are super active, an extra snack is likely needed

If this seems overwhelming, consider your childhood eating habits. Unless you experienced food insecurity, you most likely ate three meals, plus snacks at school, after school, and after dinner. To recover from your eating disorder, you will want to nourish yourself similarly.

What You Should Eat

Regarding *what* to eat, you can start with whatever *you* define as a meal or a snack—this will get you moving in the right direction. We encourage you to start with foods you feel comfortable eating. These are foods about which you don't tend to have a lot of negative feelings and with which you are familiar. Hopefully, these are also foods you enjoy; however, in the initial phases of nourishing the body, food may not be enjoyable, which is perfectly okay. In times like these—when you may not feel hungry and nothing sounds good—consider viewing food as cough syrup. Sometimes we don't want to take it and it doesn't taste good, but we know it will eventually make us feel better. It is the same with food. Try to focus on foods that are accessible and don't take a lot of time or energy to plan or prepare. In this initial phase of renourishing the body, it is often helpful, necessary, and okay to rely on convenience foods. Some find it helpful to consider that a "meal" is typically bigger than a "snack," but that doesn't have to be the case for everyone. Over time, we hope to guide you toward a more complete picture of balanced meals and snacks.

Many people restrict common "fear" foods, such as sweets. Often, when we see a person who is binge eating, they have been limiting their carbohydrate intake. However, carbohydrates are an essential nutrient that supplies our body and brain with the energy they need to function properly. The body can convert carbohydrates to glucose more easily than protein or fats, so carbohydrates are ideal for meeting our energy needs throughout the day. Due to the high energy needs in the body, particularly the brain, it is best to eat carbohydrates at regular intervals. Carbohydrates can also help people maintain muscle mass by preventing protein breakdown in muscle for energy. They can keep the body hydrated and help regulate serotonin, which can impact mood and sleep. Without enough carbohydrates, you may experience symptoms of decreased energy, fatigue, difficulties concentrating, mood swings, irritability, poor sleep, and constipation, as well as binge eating. Carbohydrates are an essential part of every meal.

Why Regular Eating Is Important for Eating Disorder Recovery

When so many aspects of disordered eating symptoms focus on weight and shape concerns, why would we ask you to focus on changing your eating routines first? There are several reasons why prioritizing changes in eating early in treatment is important.

First, eating regularly provides your body with adequate nourishment. This is especially important for those who are weight suppressed, because they must consume enough food to gain weight and address any vitamin or mineral deficiencies that may be present. This can be true no matter your body size, even if you think you are eating enough. Inadequate nutrition can lead to cognitive difficulties, including problems with attention, concentration, and memory. Once you have established a more regular eating pattern, changing the way you think about your eating habits, weight, and body becomes easier. Regular eating aims to form consistent behaviors upon which recovery can build.

Second, regular eating is also important to avoid feelings of intense hunger. It provides a structure that allows you to sense and respond to hunger cues. Binge eating can be triggered when hunger between meals gets too intense. If you allow yourself to get too hungry or run at a deficit for too long, you're more likely to binge eat or feel "out of control" with food later in the day. Many people concerned about late afternoon or evening binge eating are unaware that this behavior is linked to undereating earlier in the day, especially in the morning. Eating more frequently can prevent this buildup of hunger.

Third, regular eating is essential for improving gut function. Prolonged restriction slows digestion, making it challenging to eat enough for recovery. Eating regularly throughout the day creates more opportunities to eat so that each eating occasion can be more manageable in quantity and allow for efficient gut function to resume. Many people with disordered eating struggle with digestive disorders such as gastroparesis or irritable bowel syndrome (IBS). Regular eating can decrease discomfort, early fullness, or bloating over time. Like any part of our body, our digestive system is vulnerable to weakening if we don't use it regularly.

Fourth, regular eating is also necessary is to help minimize unwanted physical symptoms such as fatigue, dizziness, feeling faint, or passing out. These symptoms are often related to low blood sugar; sometimes they are related to other secondary effects of undereating, such as low blood pressure or anemia.

And fifth, regular eating can improve mood and emotion regulation. Many with disordered eating are familiar with being "hangry"—that is, hungry and angry blended. It is common to feel more irritable, short-tempered, or agitated, or be unable to think clearly or use planning and organizing skills, when you have gone longer periods without eating.

Consider how your energy may fluctuate during the day with regular eating. Look at the energy graph below to see how Carlos maintains his energy levels throughout the day. What might happen to his energy levels if he skips a meal or snack?

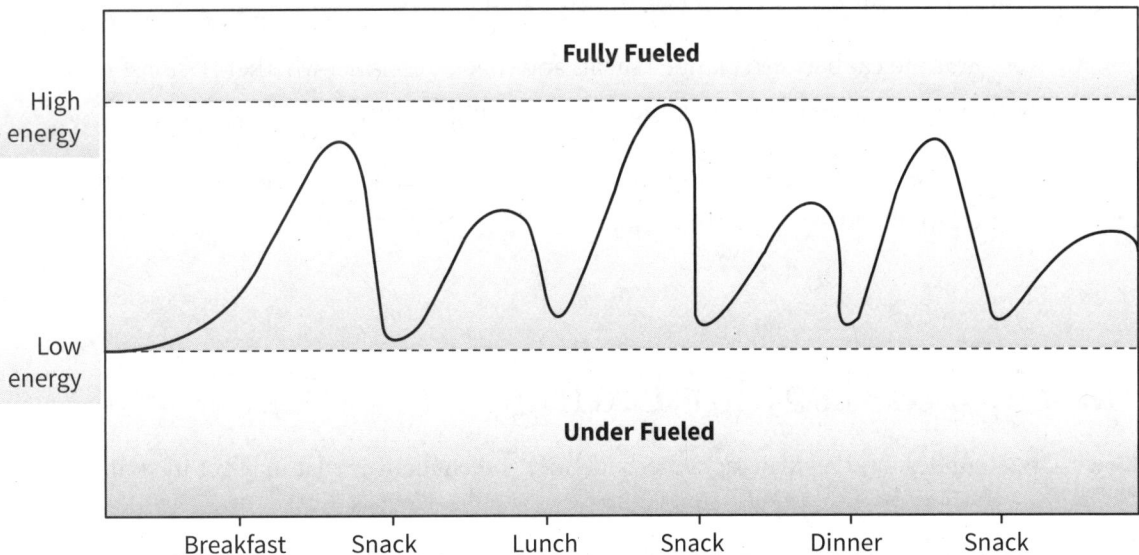

While regular eating may be hard at first—especially if you have been skipping meals or engaging in behaviors such as intermittent fasting—it becomes easier with practice and eventually becomes a habit. Over time, your body will accustom itself to eating at regular times. If managing four to six eating occasions each day feels overwhelming, start small by increasing by one eating episode per day until you feel comfortable and confident adding another.

How to Eat Regularly for Recovery

To make regular eating a priority, follow these steps:

- Start by establishing the structure and timing of meals and snacks. Later, we will help you address amount and variety.

- Plan meals or snacks in advance. Always know when and what your next meal or snack options will be. (More on this later.)

- Eat according to your schedule, regardless of whether you feel hungry.

- Set alarms to remind you to eat.

- Do not go more than four hours without eating.

- Carry snacks with you if you'll be away from home, or keep them at your workplace.

- Consider obtaining a cooler to keep in the car, if needed.

- If you want to eat between planned meals and snacks, consider whether your last meal or snack was insufficient, and adjust accordingly going forward.

- If you binge or purge, get back on track with the next scheduled mealtime (you may be tempted to skip it—but don't!).

Barriers to Regular Eating

Now that you understand regular eating, let's identify the challenges that may get in your way.

Limited Access to Foods

You may have financial or environmental barriers to getting enough food. If you feel comfortable seeking help, consider public assistance programs such as the Supplemental Nutrition Assistance Program (SNAP) and community-level programs such as food pantries and community gardens. Prioritize your recovery over any embarrassment you feel about needing assistance. If you're unsure where to start, health care providers or your local hospital can share where to access food locally. See the online resources for assistance and free food at the state and national level at http://newharbinger.com/56456.

Worries About Weight Gain

It's normal to fear regular eating when it is new to you. Many people worry they will end up "eating too much" or "not be able to stop eating" if they eat more frequently or start eating earlier in the day. Maybe you have been restricting your food intake—or believing you should—for years. Like tire tread marks in mud or ski and sledding paths at a local park in winter, our habits become deeply carved into our lives. It can be hard to escape once we fall into a restriction rut. Every time you eat regularly—even just one more meal and snack than you're used to having—your brain begins to build a new behavioral path, and it gets easier to step out of those well-worn pathways of habit.

Consider this: If regular eating leads to weight gain, your weight was probably suppressed below your body's set point, and you needed to gain that weight. While gaining weight can be scary, it can reduce your preoccupation with food, improve your health, and often improve your life. We will share resources later in this workbook to help you address fears and concerns related to weight gain. For now, establishing a regular eating pattern is one of the most effective ways to improve your symptoms. Also consider: If what you were doing before was working, would you be reading this book now?

Lack of Hunger or Desire to Eat Intuitively

We have noticed that "not being hungry" is often a barrier to regular eating. Many people have been taught to eat intuitively, relying on their body to tell them when they are hungry. This can be helpful, but early on in recovery, many people lack accurate hunger cues. Years of dieting and disordered eating dull hunger. If you have ADHD, autism, and or ARFID, you may have greater difficulty recognizing internal body sensations and processes such as hunger, thirst, and fullness. You may also forget to eat due to hyperfocus on a task of interest or a differing awareness of time. You might also struggle with organizing or preparing multistep meals.

If you have undergone bariatric surgery in the past, you may have experienced changes in your hunger and fullness cues. People taking weight loss medications (including GLP-1 agonists) or stimulant medications for ADHD or binge eating may also experience dulled hunger cues. For these and other reasons, early on in recovery, regular eating takes precedence over "intuitive eating" or "eating when hungry." Instead of asking yourself, "Am I hungry?" it is important to ask yourself, "Is it time to eat?"

Eating in public settings can be a barrier for some people. If this describes you, please see the online content, Eating in Public Settings, for more information. Similarly, grazing—eating small amounts throughout the day—can also prevent you from recognizing hunger and fullness cues. Please see the online content, Grazing.

Some people may never be able to eat according to hunger and fullness cues, and that's okay. Eating by the clock rather than waiting for hunger can help ensure you eat enough.

Digestive System Symptoms

When a person doesn't eat enough, digestion has typically slowed down, a symptom called "gastroparesis." When you start to eat more regularly for recovery, you may start to notice symptoms such as early fullness, bloating, abdominal pain, nausea, constipation, and even vomiting (Gaudiani 2019). It is important to continue eating regularly and allow your body to heal. A heating pad on the belly can provide comfort. You can also talk to your medical provider to explore physical causes or a registered dietitian to explore foods that will be better tolerated. They may recommend strategies such as increasing liquids, adding nutritional shakes, or limiting fruits and vegetables if you are experiencing bloating and fullness.

Differences in Planning, Organization, and Concentration

Some people may have difficulties with regular eating due to differences in planning, organization, attention, and concentration. If you experience any of these challenges, these strategies may be helpful. You can also check out the online content, More Meal Preparation Tips.

- Ask for help from a friend, family member, or other support person with planning, scheduling, and reminders about when to eat.

- Set alarms throughout the day on your phone based on your planned eating occasions.

- Place reminders at locations you might be during the day when it is time to eat.

- If you spend a lot of time on your computer during the day, schedule reminders on your calendar to pop up when it's close to your time to eat.

- If you find it easy to ignore alarms or reminders on your phone or computer, consider setting a timer on your microwave or oven in the kitchen. This may also help you shift from a task you are working on to eating once you are in the kitchen.

Use the following worksheet (also available online) to anticipate barriers you may have to regular eating and troubleshoot solutions.

Identify Your Barriers and Brainstorm Solutions

Barriers	Circumstances	Possible Solutions

Regular Eating Plan

Now that you understand the importance of regular eating, it's time to make your plan. Think about your day and plan the times you will eat meals and snacks. We suggest having a snack between meals that fall more than four hours apart. You don't need to be rigid about this; if you can't eat at the scheduled time, just do your best to plan on either side.

Use the following worksheet (also available online) to write out what your regular eating plan might look like. We provide an example to start.

Regular Eating Plan Example

Wakeup time: 6 a.m.

Meal / Snack	Time	Meal Plan	Notes
Breakfast	6:30 a.m.	Tortilla, eggs, bacon, and coffee	Home
Snack	10:00 a.m.	Yogurt with granola, coffee	At work
Lunch	1:00 p.m.	Pick up lunch from Subway or El Pollo Loco or bring leftovers from home	Two restaurants near office, have usuals
Snack	3:00–4:00 p.m.	Chips or cookies	Options in break room
Dinner	6:30 p.m.	Usually make dinner unless I go out	Home
Snack	9:00 p.m.	Various snacks at home like ice cream or cookies	Home

Regular Eating Plan

Wakeup time: _____

Meal / Snack	Time	Meal Plan	Notes

Meal Planning

Meal planning is another essential skill for people recovering from disordered eating (Fairburn 2008). Meal planning does not require advanced cooking skills, diet-like rigid prepping of meals at the beginning of the week, or a love of cooking. It's more like a flexible map. It's okay to plan your meals around foods that are already prepared or takeout.

We want to emphasize that meal planning for recovery differs from meal planning (or "prepping") for dieting. Meal planning for a diet usually focuses on restriction, including only the "healthiest foods" and never eating more than or in addition to the plan. Meal planning for recovery involves planning and having options available before hunger gets too intense, including varied and satisfying foods and the freedom to eat additional foods as desired.

Meal planning may require different pacing or tools for those living with chronic illness, neurodivergence, or food insecurity. We will provide potential modifications that may help.

Benefits of Meal Planning

As a strategy, meal planning has many benefits:

- Initiating a shopping trip with a list and a plan helps ensure you buy what you intend and don't become overwhelmed by choices. This may reduce anxiety around shopping.

- Having a plan can help reduce decision fatigue related to food choices as the week progresses.

- Meal planning is often more cost-effective than last-minute shopping decisions. It can stretch a budget further and may help with food insecurity. See our handout on Satisfying Eating on a Budget at http://newharbinger.com/56456.

- Planning can reduce the number of trips to the grocery store. The greater availability of food also increases the likelihood of sticking with regular eating.

Strategies for Meal Planning

Here are some strategies for planning your meals:

- **Make a plan for each meal each week.** Once a week, take twenty minutes to plan at least five breakfasts, lunches, and dinners. This schedule doesn't need to be set in stone—if you want to eat your Wednesday dinner on Tuesday instead, you'll still have all the ingredients on hand. If this feels too overwhelming, consider each night making a plan for the next day.

- **Itemize ingredients.** Make a list of the ingredients you need to buy to prepare the meals you plan. Include all items from your recipes or the prepared items you assemble for each meal.

- **Decide when you will go shopping.** Plan at least one large weekly shopping trip for your planned meals. You might also need one additional "fill-in" trip.

- **Don't forget about premade options.** If you can't or don't want to cook, you can plan delicious and balanced meals from the prepared sections of almost any supermarket. Microwavable meals are great options for many people who don't have time to cook or struggle with the organization required to make multistep meals. SNAP benefits may also cover these meals if you are using these resources. (Just remember, you may need to add sides, as many microwaveable meals are insufficient for most people.) Remember that you can also select premade options within recipes to shorten the time and the steps to complete the meal (e.g., precooked rice, premade crusts, and soup bases).

- **It doesn't have to be fresh.** It can be a lot of pressure to use fresh produce, which can also be costly. Many fruits and vegetables are perishable; exploring options like frozen and canned fruits and vegetables can be helpful.

- **Consider dining out or ordering.** If you will have some of your meals out or ordered in, write down in your weekly plan where you will go and what you think you will eat there.

- **Give yourself choices.** Even if you tend to eat the same thing for breakfast most days, try to have at least two different "go-to" breakfast options that you can alternate to ensure you have some variety.

- **Include snacks.** The snacks between meals are also important and should be part of your weekly plan.

- **Let yourself change your mind.** Including room for a spontaneous event or outing in your weekly plan is not only okay—it's encouraged. This is how meal planning for recovery differs from dieting!

You don't need to have a stocked kitchen to plan your meals. You can use the food that you have available and consider food assistance resources as needed. A meal plan prevents you from becoming too overwhelmed to decide what to eat and when. For example, if you come home from work exhausted, planning a full meal on the spot—let alone cooking it—may be so overwhelming that you simply decide *not* to eat. Or you might just start grazing or bingeing on snack foods from your cupboards and then become distressed about how much you unintentionally ate.

If you have already planned a meal—and perhaps even mostly prepared it—you have reduced the number of decisions you need to make and the work you need to do to ensure you are consistently nourishing your body in recovery.

Using our meal planning form, write your weekly meal plan. Additional copies are available at http://newharbinger.com/56456.

Weekly Meal Planning

Shopping List

Shopping List

Snacks

	Breakfast	Lunch	Dinner
M			
T			
W			
Th			
F			
Sa			
S			

Flexible Meal Planning

Some people prefer to be spontaneous. This is a great goal. However, in the early stages of recovery, it can be hard to overcome disordered eating without at least some planning. One strategy is to start by eating your first meal within an hour of waking up. Then, consider what you might be able to plan for your next meal or snack within the next two to three hours. Consider the following questions:

- What will I be doing in two to three hours?

- What foods will I have access to?

- Is there anything I need to pack to ensure that I eat regularly?

• Kendra's Story

Kendra, who has ADHD, is burned out from years of dieting and following the latest "plan" in an attempt to "manage her weight"—as her doctor encourages her to do—and is frustrated. She notices a pattern in her life. For about six weeks, she will strictly attempt to schedule every meal and snack in advance for the week. During this time, her binge eating will be low to nonexistent. Usually, these meals and snacks are carefully portioned and made the week in advance. She calls this the "honeymoon period" of dieting, during which she notices weight loss. Then something will happen—her child gets sick or someone at work assigns her a big project—and she will lose all sight of meal planning. She then will "fall off the wagon" and do no planning at all.

Kendra and her therapist create a plan to check her schedule each morning to see where she'll be during breakfast, lunch, and dinner and to identify accessible food. Today, she knows she will have access to the coffee shop around breakfast time and the cafeteria at work, where she can access lunch, but she may be stuck at work when dinner rolls around. As a result, she plans to bring several snacks with her for the day and a frozen meal if she can't make it home from work in time. She finds that this "planning on the fly" allows her to regularly eat more flexibly and sustainably.

Summary of Takeaways

Congratulations on finishing chapter 4. You've started some of the most important steps of CBT-WI. Here are the takeaways from this chapter.

- Regular eating and meal planning are crucial to interrupting disordered eating.

- Carbohydrates are villainized, but essential in your recovery.

- There are ways to overcome barriers to regular eating and meal planning.

Reflection

What are your takeaways from chapter 4? Take a moment to reflect on anything that surprised you or aspects of the chapter that felt relevant. What feelings or thoughts came up as you read the information?

_____

_____

_____

_____

_____

When to Move on to Chapter 5

- You've started to eat more consistently.

- You've used some of the tools for meal planning.

"Overeating," Undereating, "Undoing" Eating Behaviors, and Shame

Welcome to chapter 5! In chapter 4, you learned how to use regular eating and meal planning to help you recover from disordered eating. People are often hesitant about trying these strategies when they first begin treatment.

This chapter will discuss the various types of "overeating" and how restriction fuels these behaviors. You'll learn several important recovery strategies and be able to apply this information to your self-monitoring practice, gaining insight into your behaviors. If you feel overwhelmed at any point, feel free to pause and spend extra time reflecting and applying the strategies you've read about before moving forward. Recovery takes time and isn't always linear. It's normal for your motivation to go up and down as you progress through the workbook. It's also normal to slip back into old habits.

This chapter will also introduce the topic of shame related to eating behaviors. Shame doesn't start with you. It's created and reinforced by a culture that punishes fatness, disability, and differences. We've been taught to feel shame. We will show you how self-compassion can help address feelings of shame.

Reflection on Meal Planning and Regular Eating

We want to offer you an opportunity to reflect on your first few weeks of meal planning and regular eating. To do this, it might be helpful to complete the following tracker (also available online) beginning once now and then once every subsequent week.

Weekly Progress Tracker 1

Week of: _____

Review your self-monitoring records and fill in the information.

	Day 1	Day 2	Day 3	Day 4	Day 5	Day 6	Day 7
Eating Routines							
Ate breakfast							
Ate lunch							
Ate dinner							
Ate snacks							
Ate every 2–4 hours							

Once you have completed your tracker, think about any patterns you notice. Can you identify any barriers that may be hindering your regular eating progress?

_____

_____

How can you address this over the next week?

_____

_____

"Overeating"

One of the common disordered eating symptoms that people experience is "overeating." You may wonder why we have put quotes around "overeating" throughout this section. In many cases, what we find is that people's "overeating" can be more accurately understood as "rebound eating" after undereating. This is the body's attempt to make up for food you may have missed earlier in the day, week, month, or even longer due to undereating.

It is very normal to experience what many consider "overeating." Still, some people may start to experience this more often or worry that what they are experiencing goes beyond having a large portion or going back for seconds of a favorite food. Is it "overeating"? "Emotional eating"? Binge eating? How do we distinguish between these behaviors?

The amount of food matters less than the distress you might feel about these behaviors (Brownstone and Bardone-Cone 2021). Feeling out of control with food can feel scary and deserving of attention, regardless of how much you eat. So, instead of worrying too much about the quantity of food and whether it "counts" as a binge, we encourage you to consider the questions below.

What Is a Binge?

You might wonder how to tell the difference between "overeating" and a binge episode. Overeating is a subjective experience and varies greatly. A binge is a clinically defined term that describes eating what most people would describe as an "unusually large amount of food." This can be hard to quantify and varies from person to person. The criteria for binge eating suggest that most episodes last for no more than two hours, and many people describe binge episodes as happening in an even shorter time frame.

Use the following worksheet to help you determine whether you are experiencing binge-like episodes.

Exploring Binge Eating

	Yes	No
Do you feel out of control while eating? This is one of the most common signs of binge-eating behavior. You may feel as if you cannot stop eating, are not fully aware of what you are eating, or are not tasting or experiencing the food. Some people describe it as feeling like they are in a trance or rolling down a hill with such momentum that they'll keep going unless they are physically stopped.	Yes	No
Are you eating more quickly than usual?	Yes	No
Do you notice that you feel pressured to finish your food as fast as possible?	Yes	No
Do you taste your food?	Yes	No
Are you eating to the point of feeling physically uncomfortable? Although discomfort can occur with "overeating" many individuals with binge-eating behavior describe eating to the point of experiencing significant physical discomfort or feeling sick.	Yes	No
Are you hiding your eating from others? Sometimes, people who binge eat will engage in these eating episodes when they are alone due to feelings of shame or embarrassment. This may involve planning times to eat in secrecy when family members are out of the house, hiding foods during binge episodes, or stopping to pick up fast food to eat in the car on the way home.	Yes	No
How do you feel after binge eating? While it's common to feel some sense of regret after "overeating," individuals who experience binge episodes describe feeling more intense emotions such as shame, guilt, anxiety, or depression after a binge occurs.	Yes	No

Can you recall a time you experienced the behaviors above? What was happening?

_____

_____

_____

_____

_____

"Emotional Eating"

"Emotional eating" is often portrayed by diet culture as a negative behavior that needs to be reduced or eliminated. However, eating in response to feelings is a normal behavior to experience and should be accepted as a part of being human. What many people define as emotional eating is often a response to not eating enough. Eating in response to undereating is not "emotional eating"—it's often a rational and biological response to restriction.

Furthermore, most people experience "emotional eating" in their daily lives. Humans need food to survive, and eating is typically a pleasurable experience. Eating can generate positive emotions and is often an enjoyable, soothing, or calming experience. It is normal to include food to celebrate, as a reward, or as part of family routines or traditions. It is also acceptable to use food for comfort. As our colleagues Hilary Kinavy and Dana Sturtevant at the Center for Body Trust say, "Human beings turn toward food for comfort, soothing, or to check out sometimes. Eating can land us back in our bodies and be grounding. Food can signal a break and may be the only time you get a moment to yourself to pause and breathe and just be" (Center for Body Trust, e-newsletter, 2024).

Use the following worksheet to explore your experiences with "emotional eating."

Exploring "Emotional Eating"

Write about a time you ate for an emotional reason. Where were you? What time of day or night was it? How were you feeling? What was happening around you? Were you alone or with others? And what happened after you ate?

_____

_____

_____

_____

_____

Do you believe that eating is the only strategy that can help you to cope with stress or difficult emotions? How so?

_____

_____

_____

Do you believe that you rely on food to fall asleep at night or to cope with pain? Why? How does it help you?

_____

_____

Is eating one of the only things that makes you happy or feel other positive emotions? Why might that be?

_____

_____

_____

Even if you feel that you overuse eating as a coping strategy when you are not restricting, this does not mean you must focus on reducing "emotional eating." This can sometimes lead to restrictive behaviors that worsen symptoms over time. We first invite you to focus on the acceptance of "emotional eating." Can you welcome this as a strategy that works? And if you have used it in the past, has it been helpful? Taking this first step may allow you to feel more comfortable with "emotional eating." However, if you believe you rely too heavily on food for comfort, consider expanding your repertoire of coping strategies; see Alternative Coping Strategies in chapter 5.

Undereating

Undereating can take many forms, such as skipping meals, restricting the type of food consumed, restricting the amount of food consumed, or going long periods of time between meals and snacks.

If you notice any of the above, what leads you to undereat?

_____

_____

_____

Restriction isn't always intentional and can occur in people with food insecurity and those without meal breaks. Recall from chapter 4 that unintentional restriction can also occur in those with neurodivergence. Undereating may manifest not only as eating a low quantity of food but also as not allowing yourself to eat a variety of specific food groups or ingredients. Eating for joy and satisfaction is as important as eating for nutritional requirements.

• *Ava's Story*

Ava is a single mother in her thirties with limited income. She finds herself "overeating" the snack foods she buys for her child, especially at the beginning of every month when she gets her SNAP benefits. In therapy, Ava was asked to self-monitor her eating behaviors. Her monitoring forms showed that she ate mostly fruit for breakfast, a salad for lunch, a small dinner of protein and vegetables, and then binged on snack foods in the evening. Ava was asked to increase the size of her breakfasts and lunches and to include more food groups in her meals. She was surprised because she thought her meals were adequate and that her eating was "healthy." She was annoyed that she had to keep snack foods for her child in the home that could be tempting to her. She also believed she wasn't hungry for more than a piece of fruit and coffee in the morning.

After completing a brief nutrition screening conducted by her dietitian, Ava was referred to a monthly free food distribution program at her daughter's school. This program offered shelf-stable foods, such as grains, beans, and healthy fats, which helped Ava incorporate more carbohydrates and fats into her breakfasts and lunches. Combined with more mindful meal planning, this additional food support helped Ava extend her food resources throughout the month, addressing the common challenge of SNAP benefits running out by the third week. Ava was also able to access fresh fruits and vegetables at a discounted rate through a local farmers market incentive program that subsidizes the cost of locally grown produce.

Eventually, Ava's urge to eat large amounts of snack foods in the evening decreased. She realized that her previous breakfast was not sufficient even though she thought it was. She also learned that she was previously ignoring hunger cues and running on an energy deficit, which was driving her urge to eat snack foods both at night and at the beginning of every month. Eating regularly and accessing food resources were critical steps in her recovery.

The Restrict-Binge Cycle

While many diet companies would have us believe otherwise, undereating is not something our bodies are supposed to be able to do. Food is a basic need, and like the other four basic needs—water, sleep, air, and warmth— no human can survive without it (Kater 2012).

Our bodies evolved in an environment in which food was relatively scarce. Our earliest ancestors were hunters and gatherers. They had to prioritize food consumption above other activities to survive in such an environment. Whenever their food supply was less secure, stocking up when food *was* available ensured our species' survival. "Bingeing"—or prioritizing that there was enough energy-dense food when it became available—was not a matter of poor willpower but a perfectly normal and healthy body response to starvation. Conversely, anyone whose ancestors failed to "binge" on food when it became available—in the form of a rare animal wandering into their territory or a surplus of berries—would not have survived due to starvation. Their genes would not have been passed down (Neel 1962). Searching for the most energy-dense food when there is an eating lull is a survival mechanism that kept our ancestors alive when food was scarce. This is why people do not typically binge on carrots or lettuce (unless nothing else is available) and why you are more likely to binge on cookies, chips, or other energy-dense foods.

Thus, binge eating, or what most people consider "overeating," is the body's natural response to scarcity (or restricting). This is because when our basic need for food is unmet, we can become irritable and focused solely on trying to get that need met to the exclusion of other activities. We may also have poor concentration for other tasks. Finally, when that needed source becomes available, we indulge in a greater than "normal" amount. Your body doesn't know whether you are in a famine or dieting—all it knows is that you need access to high-energy food as soon as possible! Instead of criticizing yourself, marvel at your body's survival instinct.

Use the following worksheet to explore your experiences with the restrict-binge cycle.

Exploring Restrict-Binge Cycles

Think about times you have restricted food (dieted). Although initially you may have felt energized, proud, disciplined, or even euphoric, over time, did you start to notice more irritability or hangry feelings? Describe these feelings.

_____

_____

_____

Did you notice increased thoughts about food or difficulty concentrating? Describe what happened.

_____

_____

_____

Did you experience episodes of bingeing, unplanned eating, or grazing? What did you notice?

_____

_____

_____

If you don't identify with the above, reflect on a time when one of your other basic needs, such as sleep, was restricted. What happened the last time you were sleep-deprived?

_____

_____

Did you notice that it affected your mood or ability to concentrate the next day? What happened?

_____

_____

Did you catch up on extra sleep at the next opportunity or take a nap?

_____

_____

If none of the above apply, you can try the experiment of the "air diet" (Kater 2012). Take a straw and hold it in your mouth. Plug your nose with your fingers, as you would before jumping into the water. Breathe gently in and out through your mouth. This constricts the air going into your esophagus and simulates an air diet. Set a two-minute timer, open this book to a random page, and read. Stop the experiment at the end of two minutes and ask yourself the following questions.

Were you able to concentrate on the passage you were reading?

_____

How did you feel physically while your air was restricted?

_____

How did you feel emotionally?

_____

After you unplugged your nose, was your first breath a little bigger than usual?

_____

If you have restricted and not experienced a binge, just because it hasn't happened yet doesn't mean it won't. Your body's survival mechanism becomes more likely to override your control over time. Many people cross over from restriction to binge eating. Research shows that up to 62 percent of people with restricting-type anorexia eventually develop binge eating (Eddy et al. 2008). And once binge eating has started, the development of a restrictive-only eating disorder is much less common. In our experience, it appears that once the binge threshold has been crossed, it is harder to go back to restriction.

"Undoing" Eating Behaviors

Now that you understand how undereating drives binge eating or rebound eating, let us explain how "undoing" behaviors are connected. When people hear the term "purging," they often think about vomiting. But purging is any behavior meant to eliminate or "cancel out" food (energy) or liquid from the body. We also call these "undoing" behaviors. These may include:

- "Driven" exercise meant to offset what you've eaten or to lose weight

- Vomiting

- Misuse of laxatives, diuretics, or supplements with a laxative effect

- Fasting

- Misuse of prescription medications that impact weight

- Dehydrating experiences such as saunas and steam rooms

- Other behaviors that may "undo" eating

When people engage in these "undoing" or "compensatory" behaviors, their distress usually decreases. They typically resolve to "be better," which often translates into more dieting or restrictive eating. Most people dislike feeling guilt or shame, so it's not surprising if you engage in "undoing" behaviors to try to minimize it. And so the cycle repeats.

We think it's important to provide information about "undoing" behaviors so that you can better understand their role in maintaining disordered eating. Use the following worksheet to explore your experiences with "undoing" behaviors.

Exploring Your "Undoing" Behaviors

Think about the last time you ate something you didn't plan to eat or wished you hadn't eaten. How did you feel?

_____

_____

_____

When you experienced distressing feelings after eating, what did you do to manage them?

_____

_____

_____

Have you used any of the "undoing" behaviors mentioned above? What was your experience?

_____

_____

_____

Look at your self-monitoring from previous weeks. If you have identified episodes of bingeing or disordered eating, look back at your eating leading up to that episode. Were there missed snacks or meals? After these episodes, were there any "undoing" behaviors?

_____

_____

Pull out the symptom map that you started to draw in chapter 2. Can you complete any more of it now?

_____

_____

Many people have difficulty speaking about these symptoms to others—such as their doctors and loved ones—sometimes due to the shame associated with them. For others, the "undoing" behaviors may begin as an innocent attempt to improve health and may even be praised and, as such, reinforced by friends and family. This can make the cycle even more difficult to break.

• *Tara's Story*

Tara was fifteen when she developed Hashimoto's thyroiditis, a condition that resulted in hypothyroidism and weight gain. Concerned about her weight changes, her doctor referred her to a pediatric "fitness clinic," where Tara was encouraged to eat more fruits and vegetables, limit certain food groups, and engage in routine physical exercise to improve her health. Following recommendations from her doctor, Tara began reducing her carbohydrate intake and going for longer distance runs to lose weight. Her doctor, parents, and coaches praised her dedication to running and "self-discipline" in her attempt to "manage her weight."

As a result, Tara began to binge eat after her body was continually put into an energy deficit. Her ADHD medication also contributed to reduced hunger cues, and it became easy to go long periods without eating. To offset the energy consumed during her binges, Tara continued to run for longer distances. She felt stuck in this cycle of running and binge eating for years as she entered adulthood. Her social relationships suffered as she passed up opportunities to socialize with her friends so that she could exercise.

Finally, at age twenty-three, she started working with a therapist. Tara had never really considered herself to have an eating disorder—definitely not bulimia nervosa—because she had never made herself vomit after eating, and she was always praised for engaging in distance running.

Can you relate to Tara's relationship with exercise? For more support with exercise in eating disorder recovery, see the handout, Addressing Excessive Exercise, in the online resources.

Understanding "Undoing" Behaviors

People use these behaviors for various reasons. Below are several examples. Put a checkmark next to those that apply to you.

☐ To cancel out what you have eaten after a binge by attempting to limit weight gain/shape changes.

☐ To maintain a lower weight and avoid weight gain, regardless of the amount of food eaten, or to maintain a body shape that meets gendered appearance ideals.

☐ To regulate your nervous system. For some, it releases pressure when they are experiencing stress in their environment.

☐ Due to physical changes to the body. For example, people who have undergone bariatric surgery may be at risk due to discomfort associated with reduced stomach size (Conceição, Utzinger, and Pisetsky 2015).

☐ For punishment or self-harm purposes.

☐ To experience "euphoria" or a heightened state of arousal or well-being.

☐ Because of difficulty tolerating fullness. For many people with disordered eating, hunger and fullness cues and sensations may have changed. Smaller amounts of food may lead to more intense fullness sensations or even pain or discomfort, which you naturally want to relieve.

☐ To decrease certain emotions like anger, frustration, fear, loneliness, or sadness. Difficult emotions may be linked to other eating behaviors, such as breaking a dietary rule or in reaction to stressful life events.

☐ To allow for a temporary avoidance of uncomfortable thoughts or emotions such as anger, guilt, shame, sadness, or anxiety.

☐ _____

☐ _____

☐ _____

Reading this list can be distressing if you haven't thought much about the factors driving your "undoing" behaviors. Use the following worksheet to explore these emotions.

Understanding Your "Undoing" Behaviors

What have you noticed about your body sensations, thoughts, and emotions before, during, and after an "undoing" behavior?

Before: _____

_____

During: _____

_____

After: _____

_____

How are these "undoing" behaviors helping you?

_____

_____

How are these "undoing" behaviors harming you?

_____

_____

How might continued use of "undoing" behaviors impact your life five, ten, or twenty years into the future?

_____

_____

_____

If you are using "undoing" behaviors, what could motivate you to stop?

_____

_____

See also Common Misperceptions About "Undoing" Behaviors and Harm Reduction Strategies in the online materials at http://newharbinger.com/56456.

Alternative Coping Strategies

We introduce alternative coping strategies to reduce your reliance on "undoing" behaviors. These behaviors may help distract, soothe, or regulate your emotions and state of arousal. As you read through, circle any behaviors that appeal to you. Consider writing each one on a slip of paper and placing it in a small container with the others. When you experience an urge to engage in "undoing" behavior, you can easily select one to try. You can also try pairing some of the strategies together. Applying these skills when distress is high can require a lot of practice, but over time, you will be able to eliminate "undoing" behaviors.

Delay

Build in a pause. Set an alarm and encourage yourself to wait for increasing amounts of time.

This can be especially useful if your purging follows binge eating. Even if you do end up purging, you are training your brain to respond differently and dampening the strong connection between the binge and purging. During the pause you could self-monitor or add one of the other skills below.

Urge Surfing

When in doubt, ride it out! "Urge surf" by envisioning your urge to purge as a wave you can ride and eventually pass over.

Self-Soothe Using the Five Senses

Us the 5-4-3-2-1 technique to reconnect with your senses. Name five things you see in your surroundings, four things you can touch (and actually go ahead and touch them!), three things you can hear, two things you can smell (and actually smell them!), and one thing you can taste. Doing this activity can help shift your mind from anxiety-provoking thoughts and physical sensations to the present moment.

Diaphragmatic Breathing

Diaphragmatic breathing can stimulate your vagus nerve, producing feelings of relaxation and overall well-being. It can also help you reduce your heart rate. If you haven't been trained in diaphragmatic breathing, see our online resources.

Facial Temperature Changes

The dive response is a physiological reaction experienced by humans when they are submerged in cold water, and it stimulates the relaxation response. To create a dive response, fill cold water in a sealable bag and set it in the fridge. When you feel you need it, take it out and set the sealable bag on the bridge of your nose under your eyes. Ice packs or bags of frozen veggies can also work.

Ice, Ice Baby

Some people find it helpful to grab an ice pack or ice cubes and squeeze. Throwing ice cubes outside can also be cathartic. Just be careful not to get frostbite (and not to throw it near people or anything that could be damaged)!

Heating Pad

Use a heating pad to manage uncomfortable fullness after a binge.

Put in Physical Barriers

Leave the area where you may typically purge or put in other barriers. If you typically purge in the downstairs bathroom, for example, go outdoors or to a shared common space in your home. Or go for a walk or drive.

Stretch

Take a moment to stretch or try some gentle yoga. The online resources include some of our favorite practitioners.

Distract

Play music and dance if you want to. Play a game. Do a puzzle. Watch a show or read a book that captures your interest. Some people find it helpful to focus on a chore such as cleaning a room, finishing a work project, or doing homework. Add puzzles, word finds, or other activities that can aid in distraction to your "coping kit."

Animal Support

Cuddle or care for your pet or an animal.

Connect with Others

Purging is incompatible with spending time with others. Find someone else in your house to sit with or talk to. Call, text, or send a meme or video to someone. Even if you aren't comfortable talking about your eating disorder with another person, the act of connecting with others can distract you and help you feel less isolated and trapped in your head. It can take courage to open up to someone about your eating disorder.

Make a list of people with whom you can connect to distract you and with whom you may feel comfortable sharing your urges. Many people report that after telling a loved one about their struggles with purging, it can feel like a weight has been lifted off of their shoulders and that it becomes harder to purge without the veil of secrecy.

People I can reach out to distract myself:

_____

_____

_____

_____

People I can reach out to and share my struggles with:

_____

_____

_____

Create and Repeat a Coping Statement

Develop and practice coping statements that can help you during difficult moments. For example:

"Fullness and hard feelings always pass."

"My body knows what to do with this sensation of fullness."

"Feeling full is my body's way of creating awareness for me."

"I can tolerate what comes my way—I am safe now."

Write your coping statement down to refer to when you have an urge to purge.

_____

_____

Identify and Label Your Thoughts and Feelings

You might want to record your thoughts and feelings on your self-monitoring log or in a journal. Avoid getting "hooked" or too attached to those thoughts and feelings. Use the Feelings Wheel tool to help you identify various emotions.

Remember, You Will Get Hungry Again

Remember that regardless of how much you've eaten or how full you feel, the sensation will pass, and you will feel hungry again.

Now, take a moment to review the above list and use the worksheet, My Coping Skills Plan, to list the strategies that work best for you. Consider saving a picture of your completed coping skills plan on your phone for easy access.

My Coping Skills Plan

My favorite strategies for when I'm in public:

1. _____

2. _____

3. _____

My favorite strategies for when I'm at home alone:

1. _____

2. _____

3. _____

Caring for Yourself: Approaching Shame with Self-Compassion

We encourage you to notice and name any thoughts, emotions, or bodily sensations you are experiencing. Acknowledging the uncomfortable experiences that often come with disordered eating can be difficult. We're so proud of you for sticking with us and know that you can do the hard work of learning more about your emotions, thoughts, and behaviors!

For many, examining and sharing their eating disorder behaviors may lead them to experience shame. Hilary Kinavey and Dana Sturtevant at the Center for Body Trust so wisely describe shame as "the feeling that causes you to shrink, feel small, less significant, like hiding. Sometimes, when you have recognized the visceral reaction within that is shame, it can be startling to notice when and how often you feel it. In the body, shame often feels like a warm or hot rising feeling. It can feel like slime, lava, or ick" (Center for Body Trust, e-newsletter, 2024). As we noted previously, shame does not start with you. It is present in the culture and systems that influence how we feel about ourselves. We will discuss the complexity of these emotions as they relate to body image in chapter 7.

The remedy for shame is self-compassion, or offering kindness to ourselves (Neff and Germer 2018). Self-compassion can help support eating disorder recovery (Morgan-Lowes et al. 2023). For these reasons, we believe it's crucial to understand how your behaviors serve you and cultivate self-compassion. In other words, how is the symptom you are experiencing serving you? To answer this question, it may be helpful to return to your pros and cons of change list from chapter 1. Inviting yourself to consider ways your behaviors serve a purpose is a great start to harvesting self-compassion. It might be helpful for you to ask how you might talk to or care for a loved one in a similar situation. Then try to talk to yourself in a similar way.

Here are three additional steps that we encourage you to try as you begin a self-compassion practice:

1. Self-compassion invites you to *pause* during painful situations to take mindful notice of what you are experiencing. This might include naming and acknowledging your hurt by saying, "Ouch; that was painful" or "I'm really hurting now." Some people benefit from hugging themselves, gently touching their arms, or caressing their own faces.

2. Next, *know that you are not alone* in your struggles. Sometimes, the loneliness and shame we experience can alienate us to the point of feeling as if there is something fundamentally wrong with us. Knowing that pain and suffering are a universal human experience reminds us that it is not a personal shortcoming. It's important to note that this is not meant to invalidate or compare your struggles to others, but rather to reduce isolation and shame.

3. Finally, ask yourself *what you need at this moment* to lessen your suffering and care for yourself. If unsure, reflect on common human needs, including physical or emotional nourishment, sleep, validation or acceptance, human connection through physical touch or emotion, self-expression, or stimulation. (Hint: The coping kit you create in this chapter may offer some support with this!) If what you need isn't accessible—if a loved one isn't available to talk to or you can't safely scream it out—consider what might be doable in the moment. For example, you could journal your experience or visualize what it might feel like to meet this need in the future.

We like to gently remind people that repetitive behaviors such as bingeing or purging often serve a purpose. At the same time, they are probably not helping you as much as you think. Reframing your behaviors as an attempt to help yourself through difficult times can be the first step to offering yourself compassion. Read about the way that binge eating served Sam during difficult times.

- *Sam's Story*

Sam experienced rejection from their family when they came out as nonbinary. They often witnessed conflict between their parents. Furthermore, diet culture was prominent in Sam's family. Their sister and mom would frequently diet and hide certain foods to keep them "out of sight and out of mind." These were some of Sam's favorite foods. With the stress of rejection, parental conflict, and fighting in the evenings, Sam would often rummage the cupboards for baked goods, chips, and other snacks and retreat into their bedroom. When Sam started eating these enjoyable foods, they found that it was an opportunity to tune out the fighting and distract themselves from the stressors they faced at home and school.

During a binge, the outside yelling quieted, as did the racing thoughts Sam experienced. In therapy, Sam learned that binge eating helped them (temporarily) distract themselves from anger and sadness sparked by stressful events that occurred at home and school. Together, Sam and their therapist identified ways for them to access a self-compassion practice after binge eating and eventually before binge eating. Self-compassion allowed Sam to identify their needs and increase coping strategies. Using a cool compress on their face or hands, texting or sending funny memes to a friend on Instagram, and watching a funny show on their iPad became their go-to strategies, which allowed for connection, physiological calming, and distraction.

The Self-Compassion Practice Activity, adapted from Neff and Germer (2018), is available in the online resources.

Summary of Takeaways

Way to go! You've made it through chapter 5. Remember that we provide many resources online that you can return to during times of need. Here are some takeaways:

- "Overeating" and "emotional eating" are common experiences.

- Binge eating involves experiencing a loss of control that is often accompanied by physical discomfort, negative emotions, and a change in eating patterns, such as eating faster or eating alone due to embarrassment.

- "Overeating," "emotional eating," and binge eating often result from undereating and limiting enjoyable foods. If you're looking to reduce the occurrence of these behaviors, we recommend eating more—not less.

- "Undoing" behaviors are attempts to "cancel out" food that is eaten, and they pose health risks and continue the restrict-binge cycle.

- Eating and "undoing" behaviors described in this chapter often serve a purpose. It's important first to understand how they may be helping you to identify additional ways to cope.

- Self-compassion can be a useful way to help yourself during difficult times.

Reflection

What are your takeaways from chapter 5? Take a moment to reflect on what you learned or parts of the chapter that might be useful to review. You may consider sharing these observations if you are currently working with a therapist.

_____

_____

_____

_____

_____

When to Move on to Chapter 6

- You've completed relevant reflection questions in the chapter.

- You've created a list of coping strategies to try (even if you're not ready to use them).

Chapter 6

Eating for Recovery

In most cases, people with eating issues will need to eat more than they think they need for recovery. As we said in chapter 4, at the start of treatment you should focus mostly on the structure of regular eating. Now that you have been at it for a little while, let's review what you've noticed in your monitoring records. We'll continue our focus on when to eat and later in this chapter, we'll explore what to eat.

Review of Monitoring Records

As you move through the rest of the chapters in this book, we will ask you to review your self-monitoring record for the previous week. Think about the symptoms you have been experiencing and when they occurred over the past week. You can use the following tracker to record behaviors. Using your self-monitoring forms, complete the Weekly Progress Tracker (also available online) by indicating the number of times each behavior occurred each day.

Weekly Progress Tracker 2

	Day 1	Day 2	Day 3	Day 4	Day 5	Day 6	Day 7
Eating Routines							
Ate breakfast							
Ate lunch							
Ate dinner							
Ate snacks							
Ate every 2–4 hours							
Other Eating Behaviors							
Restriction							
Binge eating							
Self-induced vomiting							
Laxative use							
Excessive exercise or movement							
Excessive water or caffeine							
Other behaviors (e.g., chewing and spitting, using saunas, etc.)							

After completing this tracker, what do you notice?

_____

_____

_____

Based on your observations above, what goals, if any, would you like to set for the next week?

1. _____

2. _____

3. _____

4. _____

5. _____

6. _____

Improving Volume: Are You Eating Enough?

Most of the time, people with disordered eating need to eat more. It's okay if you don't believe that—diet culture can be subtle and seductive. Take the following quiz (also available online) to determine whether you are eating enough.

Quiz: Are You Eating Enough?

Look at your self-monitoring forms and circle your answers below.

Did you eat at least three meals and two snacks per day most days?	**YES**	NO
Did you have gaps greater than four hours between meals and snacks?	YES	**NO**
Did you think about food often between meals?	YES	**NO**
Did you have intense food cravings?	YES	**NO**
Did you have decreased ability to concentrate on tasks?	YES	**NO**
Did you feel satisfied at the end of most meals and snacks?	**YES**	NO
Did you feel your meals and snacks "held you" until the next meal or snack?	**YES**	NO
Did you get irritable or "hangry" in the afternoon or evening?	YES	**NO**
Did you have stable energy levels throughout the day?	**YES**	NO

Did you have any episodes of bingeing or unplanned eating?	YES	**NO**
Did you have restful sleep?	**YES**	NO
Did you have regular digestion and bowel movements?	**YES**	NO

If you chose the unbolded answers to any of these questions, identify below a goal you can set for the next week to address this. For example, do you need to add more snacks? Do you need to add more items to your meals? Do you need to increase the size of your meals? If you selected many unbolded answers, it's okay to start with one goal.

If you answered mostly the bolded items, great job! Is there anywhere you could still make changes?

Write out your "eating enough" goal:

_____

_____

If you are weight suppressed, meaning you have lost weight due to your eating disorder, you must ensure you are eating sufficiently. This likely means that you will gain weight, which is exactly what your body needs to do. To make this happen, we encourage you to work on gradually increasing the volume and density of foods you eat. If you are in a higher weight body, you will likely need even more food, not less, contrary to mainstream advice (Lazzer et al. 2007). Don't be fooled by the very low-calorie goals promoted by some weight loss programs. They often do not have enough food to sustain even a child.

Common Experiences with Regular Eating

Below, we'll describe common experiences with regular eating and strategies to manage them.

Early Fullness

As we have already discussed, early fullness is common (see chapter 4). Eating denser foods—that is, foods with more calories and less volume—and liquid calories can help if you are experiencing this symptom. These might include peanut butter, avocado, cheese, ice cream, and butter. Of course, you should consult a medical doctor if you are experiencing significant pain.

Extreme Hunger

Some people recovering from eating disorders experience extreme hunger once they start eating again. This hunger can be frightening and can sometimes result in binge eating. If you've been feeling this, we want to reassure you that this is your body's way of helping you to eat more. It does not mean your body is broken, and you will not keep eating like this for a lifetime. The best way to address extreme hunger is to maintain regular and sufficient eating behavior so that your body grows to learn and trust that it will continue to be fed.

Recognizing Hunger and Fullness Cues

If you are not experiencing early fullness with regular eating, we recommend using the Hunger-Fullness Scale (Craighead 2006) to help you increase awareness of hunger cues.

1	2	3	4	5	6	7
Too hungry		Neither hungry nor full			So uncomfortably full	

If you think of your sense of fullness as a pendulum that swings on this scale, you want to control how far it swings. You do not want to swing wildly between 1 and 7—letting your "gas tank" get totally empty before refilling to the bursting point. You want to stay in the middle, fluctuating primarily within the shaded area, about 2.5 to 5.5. This may mean unlearning some lessons you have learned from diet culture, such as "I should only eat when I am hungry," and standing up to eating disorder rules, such as "I only deserve to eat if I get to the point of starving." Similarly, many people fear feeling full. We want to remind you that fullness is your body's signal to stop eating. Becoming full is the goal, not something to be feared.

Ideally, you want to begin eating before you get below a 2 on the scale, and each time you eat, you want to cross the midline (4) and get to a 5 or higher. Eating every three hours should help hold you if your meals and snacks are adequate in volume. We acknowledge that this might be challenging if you have issues with food accessibility. You may not have full control over when you can eat.

We also want to reassure you that there is no problem with getting to a 6 or 7. Diet culture will tell you this is bad. We disagree. However, we know that the intense distress many people feel when they get to a 6 or 7 may drive them to use an "undoing" behavior. You are more likely to swing to a 6 or 7 when you've fallen to a 1 or 2.

If hunger cues are not accessible to you at this point, you may want to continue to focus on regular eating and plan to revisit this section later. It's also important to know that for some people, hunger cues can continue to be difficult to identify. That's okay, too; see the sidebar that follows for hunger cues.

We suggest that this week, you incorporate your hunger and fullness ratings at each eating episode in your self-monitoring record. We've provided a new self-monitoring form in the online resources that includes a column to record your rating. You should try to have a different rating before and after eating—to reflect this, just put the two numbers in the box, i.e., "2 / 5.5" or "3 / 6."

When done together with regular eating, checking in on your hunger-fullness levels before you begin eating and after you finish can help:

- Increase your awareness of hunger and fullness cues

- Ensure meals are timed correctly

- Ensure meals suffice to hold you to the next eating opportunity

- Identify when an urge to eat might signal a different unmet need

For example, if you eat breakfast at 7 a.m. but find you're hungry at 9 a.m.—an hour before your planned 10 a.m. snack—what are your options? You can have your snack earlier, add an extra snack, or wait it out. But you should also consider what else this feedback may indicate. Was your breakfast too small? Is 10 a.m. the best time for a snack, or should you plan to snack at 9 a.m.? Or were you just unusually hungry today? It's normal for the amount of food you need to vary. Some days, you may be hungrier than others. It may be that you were more active or slept less. Often, there may be no clear reason. Don't be overly rigid about staying in the sweet spot of the continuum between hunger and fullness. This is just a tool to use alongside regular eating—not an excuse to delay eating until you reach the "right hunger level" or to reinforce restriction.

Finally, for anyone who struggles to record foods eaten in their self-monitoring forms, we offer this alternative: keep your hunger and fullness ratings and times of eating in the last column only, and don't complete the food intake column. This simpler data will still provide helpful information (Craighead 2006).

Hunger Signs

The only hunger sign some people may be attuned to is a rumbling in their stomachs. But this is usually one of the later hunger signals—it may be a sign that you've waited far too long to eat. Below is a list, reprinted by permission of Seven Health Eating Disorder Recovery and Anti-Diet Nutritionist, of other thoughts, feelings, and sensations that may be more subtle signs of hunger. Many of them can occur for reasons other than hunger as well, so if you experience any of them, you should try to notice whether they seem to be connected to your eating.

- Feeling of emptiness in stomach
- Gurgling, rumbling, or growling in stomach
- Thoughts about food
- Dizziness, faintness, or lightheadedness
- Headache
- Fatigue—a weak, tired, or shaky feeling
- Daytime sleepiness
- Irritability or easily agitated
- Lack of concentration
- Indecisiveness
- Nausea or "car sickness" feeling
- Acid reflux
- Increased thirst or dry mouth
- Frequent urination, especially if clear
- Cold hands, feet, or tip of the nose
- Blurred vision, straining eyes, or vision changes
- Anxiety
- Nervousness
- Heart palpitations
- Low mood
- Anger and frustration

"Food Noise"

With the advent of GLP-1 weight loss medications, we have observed that hunger cues can be misconstrued or pathologized as "food noise." We want to emphasize that we commonly see people with eating issues who are preoccupied with food, thoughts of food, and what their next meal or snack should or shouldn't be. These hunger cues and preoccupation are symptoms of dietary restriction and usually improve or go away when people increase the frequency and volume of their eating. In fact, we want you to tune in to the food noise—this music is probably playing for a reason—and nourish yourself accordingly rather than drowning out your hunger cues. You may be thinking, "But if I listen to this food noise, I'll never stop eating!" We encourage you to be patient and see how this shifts with ongoing progress with regular and sufficient eating.

• Alberto's Story

Alberto sought treatment for "emotional eating." His eating pattern was coffee for breakfast, a salad for lunch, and what he considered a balanced dinner: a plate of rice, broccoli, and chicken. He would occasionally have two cookies after dinner and felt guilty about this behavior.

As he worked on building regular eating habits, he focused on adding breakfast, a more substantial lunch, and an afternoon snack. At the onset, this was hard because he was not hungry for breakfast, got full very quickly, and was afraid eating more would cause weight gain.

After a few months, Alberto was introduced to the hunger-fullness scale to help fine-tune his regular eating. Alberto noticed that he was, in fact, hungry for breakfast. He also learned that thinking about food was often a sign that he was hungry and that waiting for stomach hunger and pain—1 or 2 on the scale—was often too late and led to nausea and agitation. He also learned that if he had a meeting during his regular lunchtime, he should eat earlier, even if not hungry, to avoid getting too hungry. For example, on Wednesdays, he taught a class that started at 12 p.m. and did not have a break until 4 p.m. Eating lunch at 11 a.m. and a quick snack during class break at 2 p.m. allowed him to stay fully fueled for the afternoon. Over time, Alberto noticed more energy throughout the day, and he no longer felt guilty about enjoying cookies.

Expanding Your Variety of Foods

Once you feel more comfortable with eating enough for recovery, you should consider ways to increase variety in your food choices. Your recent experience with eating may have focused mainly on restricting or limiting calories, carbohydrates, or certain food groups. Switching your focus to eating a wider variety of foods again may be difficult at first but it will become more rewarding over time.

> Take a moment to reflect on the foods that you've recorded on your self-monitoring forms. Are there food groups you don't include that you enjoy or miss? Are there foods that your family or members of your peer group eat that you don't?
>
> _____
>
> _____
>
> _____
>
> _____
>
> _____
>
> _____

What Should You Eat?

This can be a great time to reach out for support from a registered dietitian. Getting enough food and ensuring that you consume a variety of nutrients helps your body function properly throughout the day. For some, this process can create anxiety. You may worry about eating foods you were previously told to avoid, such as carbohydrates or fats. Rest assured—this type of eating does not involve any restriction. It focuses on adding in more foods to make sure your nutritional needs are being met.

A simple way to begin is to consider what nutrients everyone needs to survive and foods in which you can find them. These can also be considered essential elements that our body cannot produce on its own:

- Water

- Carbohydrates/starches—bread, pasta, cereal, rice, sweets

- Protein—meat, fish, beans, tofu, dairy, nuts

- Fat—oil, butter, avocado

- Vitamins/minerals—found in fruits, vegetables, whole grains

When people limit their food choices, they may notice increased cravings for those foods at other times of the day. They might also notice that they feel hungry frequently or never feel satisfied. For example, someone limiting carbohydrates throughout the day may eat more than planned at night of mostly carb-heavy foods. Or someone unaware that their meals and snacks throughout the day lack protein may feel unsatisfied and find themselves grazing for several hours in the afternoon or evening. Eating the full range of the above nutrients regularly can help you feel full and satisfied.

Considering how to incorporate all these different types of food can be overwhelming. The following worksheet (also available online) will help you simplify this process.

Eating for Recovery

First, consider your current eating routine and what you typically have at different meals and snacks throughout the day. Which of the above categories do you feel like you are eating already?

_____

_____

Which categories might be missing from your current routine? Are there certain meals or snacks that tend to be more balanced than others?

_____

_____

What types of foods do you enjoy in the missing categories? Are there foods that would be convenient to add to your routine?

_____

_____

Do you face any barriers to getting certain categories of food?

_____

_____

Finally, think about a few simple changes you can make to start incorporating the foods you identified above. Are there one or two changes you would feel comfortable making over the next week?

_____

_____

Remember, the goal here is more flexibility, not rigidity. Start small with one or two additions a week. See how you feel after making these changes. Keep in mind it's normal to have meals and snacks that do not have all these categories, and that's okay. If you do not have access to a dietitian and would like more guidance in this area, consider the book *How to Nourish Yourself Through an Eating Disorder* (Sterling and Crosbie 2023).

A Note on Food Insecurity

Increasing variety can be especially challenging for people who do not have consistent access to food or certain types of foods. For example, some people may not easily access fresh fruits and vegetables or protein sources. Some people seeking eating disorder treatment may feel discouraged when they are not able to follow a meal plan or eating routine recommended by their treatment team (Hazzard et al. 2020). If you take medications, affording both medications and an adequate amount of food may be challenging.

If you experience food insecurity, we recommend you focus first on regular eating and work on expanding variety later. You can identify potential gaps and consider ways to address them in the future if it is not possible now. If access to fresh food is limited, remember that frozen and canned fruits and vegetables provide similar vitamins and minerals. Canned meats such as chicken and tuna can also be great protein sources. Consider food resources available in your community as well. In the online resources, we have noted some national organizations and suggested where to look for similar programs locally.

Finally—just do your best! Eating a variety of foods is challenging even for those with more consistent access to food. Give yourself time and space to make these changes slowly so that this area does not add more pressure or stress.

Sensory Differences

If you experience difficulties with specific tastes, textures, or other food characteristics, reconnecting with the experience of eating and incorporating new or different foods may create anxiety and stress. Consider this: There are no right or wrong foods in the categories listed above. Find an option that works for you and stick with it for now. You can always experiment with adding new foods later—but right now, the overall focus is on getting a wider variety of foods. You do not need to include foods that create uncomfortable sensory experiences. For example, if you know that vegetables and fruits typically challenge you more, do not feel pressured to add them. We recommend seeking help from a registered dietitian who has experience working with people who have sensory differences. They may also be able to recommend supplements to balance any nutritional deficiencies you may experience.

Reconnecting with the Experience of Eating

Many people find that they do not spend much time on their meals and snacks throughout the day or feel rushed or distracted while they are eating. As you incorporate a more consistent eating routine and add variety to your foods, consider how to carve out time to feel present while eating. At first, this may feel uncomfortable. You may notice boredom, anxiety, or restlessness while you are eating. Take your time and focus on what you experience with your food. The following worksheet (also available online) will help you explore your usual eating routine.

Eating Awareness

Do you set aside enough time to enjoy your meals and snacks? How much time do you typically have to eat your food?

_____

Do you tend to multitask when you are eating? Maybe you sit at the computer, watch TV, or scroll on your phone? What do you notice about your eating when you are doing two things at once?

_____

_____

How much do you engage your other senses when you are eating? Do you tend to notice how your food looks or smells before eating it? If you do, does that make your eating experience more enjoyable?

_____

_____

Here's another way to explore your awareness when it comes to eating: Choose a food that you enjoy and feel comfortable eating. Set aside five minutes without distractions to fully focus on eating. First, take a few moments to look at the food and describe any thoughts, feelings, or physical sensations that arise as you think about eating it. As you take the first few bites, notice any additional reactions or sensations. Observe what tastes and flavors you enjoy and what other aspects of eating you find pleasurable.

Write your thoughts about the above activity and what you noticed.

_____

_____

_____

These strategies may also help you identify which foods you find most satisfying and enjoyable as you expand your variety.

Diet Culture, Eating Rules, and Avoided Foods

Recall how we defined diet culture in the introduction: a societal system that values people based on their appearance, especially their body size and shape. Eating rules loom large in diet culture. You can think of eating rules as the wires that make up the cage of diet culture. These rules are strict, self-identified guidelines about food and eating. Most eating rules are inflexible and rooted in "all-or-nothing" thinking. In other words, if the rule is not followed exactly, it is considered broken. These rules often come in four main forms: *how* to eat, *how much* to eat, *when* to eat, and *what* to eat. Use the following worksheet to explore your eating rules.

Eating "Rules"

Examples of rules about *how to* eat:

- I have to eat slowly.

- I have to chew food a specific number of times.

- I have to eat certain food groups first before others.

Circle any of the above rules that apply to you. Add any additional food rules that you have about how to eat below.

_____

_____

_____

Examples of rules about *how much* to eat:

- I will have one serving of a "treat" per day.

- I will keep within a certain carbohydrate limit daily.

- I have to limit myself to one serving size of a food.

- I have to eat less than others around me.

Circle any of the above rules that apply to you. Add any additional food rules that you have about how much to eat below.

_____

_____

_____

Examples of rules that involve *when* to eat:

- I will not eat after 7 p.m.

- I won't eat until dinnertime.

- If I'm not experiencing hunger cues, I shouldn't eat.

Circle any of the above rules that apply to you. Add any additional food rules that you have about when to eat below.

_____

_____

_____

Examples of rules about *what* to eat (or not eat):

- I can only have one type of carbohydrate per meal.

- I have to eat a vegetable at every meal.

- I can only have fast food once per month.

Circle any of the above rules that apply to you. Record any additional rules that you have about what to eat below. If you find yourself listing specific foods that you consider off-limits, hold off for a moment! You will list those in the next activity.

_____

_____

_____

How easy was it to list your eating rules? You might feel overwhelmed by the number of rules that you identified. You might have even lacked the space to list all of them. You might have also had difficulty identifying any food rules. Many people find that their food rules have become so commonplace after a lifetime of dieting that they don't think twice about them or even recognize them as a rule.

Sometimes rules about eating have been recommended to you by medical professionals to manage a condition such as diabetes. We acknowledge that differentiating between the two can be tough. See the online content, Medical Guidelines vs. Eating Rules.

Breaking the Rules

After you've listed your eating rules, predict what you think might happen if you break them. Then test those predictions with behavioral experiments to see whether your predictions about feared events come true. This also trains you to tolerate the uncertainty of not knowing the outcome.

You've probably heard the phrase "you don't know until you try." This is the spirit of a behavioral experiment. Like scientists testing hypotheses, we want to invite curiosity to see whether our predictions are accurate. In addition to identifying your rules and fears about breaking them, we also think it's essential to identify their origins, how they might be serving you—or not—and reasons to break them. Maria's story offers an example.

• Maria's Story

Maria has a history of breast cancer and was advised to "maintain her weight" after she received her diagnosis and treatment. As you read Maria's example worksheet, we encourage you to complete this activity using one of your own rules from the previous worksheet. A blank worksheet follows Maria's example, and it can also be found online.

Breaking the Rules Worksheet, Maria's Example

Step 1: Identify the food rule or avoided eating situation.

"I should avoid all processed foods and eat only 'whole foods.'"

Step 2: Reflect on where you learned the rule.

After receiving my chemotherapy treatment, my doctor referred me to a lifestyle change program. I was told in the program that I should avoid foods that are packaged and processed and instead eat only fresh produce, whole grains, and small amounts of lean protein. I also see a lot of articles in the news about "ultra-processed" foods being bad for me.

Step 3: Ask yourself, "How is this rule working for me?" List the upsides and downsides of the rule.

Although I notice a positive impact on my digestion and feel proud of myself when I avoid processed foods, I also feel deprived when I cut them out. It's hard to find anything to eat when I go out with my friends for dinner, so I avoid spending time with people. Avoiding all processed foods also means that I spend a lot more time cooking and preparing my food, which isn't realistic given my current schedule. I also feel very out of control around these foods when I have access to them. Most importantly, it's really expensive to follow a "whole foods" diet.

Step 4: Reframe the food rule based on past experience and new information.

My past experiences show that when I don't eat processed foods, I end up feeling deprived, tired from cooking all the time, and have expensive grocery bills. I also feel guilty when I break this rule, which makes me feel bad about myself. My dietitian tells me that it's not realistic to avoid all processed foods. Some of what I learned in the lifestyle program may not be supported by strong research studies.

Step 5: Identify ways to break the food rule and why it's important to break it.

I will incorporate processed foods with at least two meals and one snack during the day for one week. This is important for me to try because I'd like to spend more of my life doing things that matter more to me—such as spending time with my family—and spend less time stressing about food.

Step 6: Reflect on your experience after breaking the rule (if you wish, you can use a scale of 1 to 10 to rate your anxiety). Did your feared prediction(s) come true? If so, how did you cope? Did you tolerate the uncertainty of not knowing?

At first, I felt guilty when I started eating processed foods again, but this lessened over time. My anxiety was about an 8 out of 10 the first time I ate processed food and about 2 out of 10 during the most recent time. Eating with others helped. I didn't notice any changes in my digestion in the ways that I thought. Breaking this rule helped me feel less out of control around these foods and allowed me to have time and energy to pursue other activities in my life, like caring for my granddaughter and spending time with friends. While I don't know for sure whether my cancer will come back, I can tolerate that uncertainty. I know I am trying to be consistent with follow-up medical care that is important for my health.

Breaking the Rules Worksheet

Step 1: Identify the food rule or avoided eating situation.

_____

_____

Step 2: Reflect on where you learned the rule.

_____

_____

Step 3: Ask yourself, "How is this rule working for me?" List the upsides and downsides of the rule.

_____

_____

_____

_____

Step 4: Reframe the food rule based on past experience and new information.

_____

_____

_____

_____

Step 5: Identify ways to break the food rule and why it's important to break it.

_____

_____

_____

_____

_____

Step 6: Reflect on your experience after breaking the rule (if you wish, you can use a scale of 1 to 10 to rate your anxiety). Did your feared prediction(s) come true? If so, how did you cope? Did you tolerate the uncertainty of not knowing?

_____

_____

_____

_____

_____

Identifying Avoided Foods

Some people experience *intense* fears associated with eating specific foods. At the same time, others describe foods as being too "tempting" or "challenging" to have around the house because they may binge or lose control when eating them. Often, we hear the term "junk food" to describe these specific foods. Regardless of your experience, food and eating-related avoidance maintains disordered eating (Christian and Levinson 2022). In this section, you'll learn how to incorporate avoided foods with behavioral experiments. Over time, this can help you feel more comfortable with these foods.

If you find yourself labeling certain foods as "junk," "sinful," "bad," or any other negative descriptor, what impact do you think this has on your relationship with these foods?

_____

_____

_____

_____

As previously discussed, we know that each food group has a function. Consider neutralizing your description of foods first. Rather than classifying the food as "healthy" or "unhealthy," it may help to identify what nutrients the food provides. For example, some types of pizza may have carbohydrates (crust), protein (cheese), fat (pepperoni), and fiber (vegetable toppings).

You may find that you've gotten a lot of advice on what foods to eat or avoid. This is especially true if you've had the experience of dieting or being told to "manage" your weight from a young age. The food that you eat starts to have a moral value and may impact your self-worth. How might changing how you describe or label foods change your experience of eating them?

_____

_____

_____

_____

Although the following adjectives are not necessarily neutral, some people have found the terms "fun" foods or "enjoyable" foods to be more helpful ways to describe foods eaten primarily for pleasure. Contrary to what diet culture would lead us to believe, our bodies can handle several cupcakes! These foods might also provide a lot of meaning and positive energy in other ways, like celebrating a birthday or making a beloved family recipe.

Identify any foods that you consider "forbidden" or that you don't allow yourself to eat. If it's helpful, you can imagine yourself walking down each aisle of your local grocery store or looking at a menu at your favorite restaurant. What foods and drinks do you see? Are there any you might enjoy eating but wouldn't buy or order? List everything that you would consider a "forbidden" food or drink. *Note that religious practices, medical food restrictions, severe allergies, and cost of foods may be valid reasons for avoiding specific foods and do not need to be included here.*

_____

_____

_____

_____

_____

_____

_____

_____

_____

_____

After you've identified the foods you're avoiding, use the following worksheet (also available online) to separate them by the degree to which you fear reincorporating them. You may already be eating these foods during binge episodes but are still trying to avoid them in other situations. In these cases, you may still feel scared or anxious about incorporating the foods into your usual meals and snacks.

Reincorporating Avoided Foods

When you think about the foods you're avoiding, how much do you fear reincorporating them?

Slightly Scary	Medium Scary	Super Scary

After listing and categorizing your avoided foods, we invite you to select one or two to incorporate into your meals and snacks over the next week. You may choose to "go low and slow" by selecting items from the left-hand column. Alternatively, you could choose to dive right in and try foods that are more challenging for you. The beauty of this design is that you get to choose where you start.

How to Set Yourself Up for Success

When first incorporating avoided foods, planning ahead is helpful to ensure you are prepared for the experience. For example, if pizza is one of your scariest, most avoided foods, we would not recommend ordering a pizza when you're home alone after not eating much during the day. Instead, try an outing with a friend for pizza where you can order a few slices or share a pizza. Make sure you are eating regularly and avoiding restriction in the days leading up to and after your planned avoided foods experiments. The goal is to do the exposure and not use an "undoing" behavior after. You can use the coping strategies you identified in chapter 5. To get the most out of the process, we encourage you to complete the following worksheet (also available online) each time you try a new food.

Incorporating Avoided Foods Reflection

Date: _____

The food I incorporated: _____

Where and when I ate it—setting, location, situation: _____

_____

Who I was with: _____

Rate your distress on a scale of 1 to 10, with 1 being not at all distressed to 10 being very distressed.

Before eating the food: _____

While eating the food: _____

After eating the food: _____

What were you afraid might happen if you ate this food? What made it difficult?

_____

_____

_____

Did your fear come true?   ☐ Yes   ☐ No

If so, how did you cope with it?

_____

_____

_____

How was the outcome different from what you expected? What surprised you about the outcome and what did you learn?

_____

_____

_____

When will you do this experiment again? _____

How can you increase your level of difficulty? If this felt too difficult or you had a hard time coping, can you change anything about your surroundings or support to make it easier?

_____

_____

We know that asking you to break your food and eating rules can be scary. But you should know that breaking the rules is rooted in a type of therapy called exposure therapy, which is used in the treatment of anxiety and eating disorders (Butler and Heimberg 2020). The more you expose yourself to something you fear, the less scary it becomes. You learn that you can tolerate facing those fears and the uncertainty of the outcome.

You might identify with feeling "addicted" to certain foods. If this sounds like you, see Are You Addicted to Food? in the online resources.

Eating with Permission and Honoring Your Taste Preferences

One of the most difficult yet necessary parts of healing your relationship with food might be to honor your true taste preferences. For so many reasons, this process can be difficult. You might have been told that your taste preferences are "wrong" somehow or that your culturally preferred foods are "unhealthy." Others have described growing up in a household with "healthy" versions of commonly enjoyed foods that never satisfied them.

Take a moment to reflect on some of your favorite foods. What makes them your favorite? Do particular flavors, textures, temperatures, or presentation styles attract you? These might be foods you used to enjoy (perhaps as a child) but no longer allow yourself to eat.

Diet culture has a sneaky way of overwriting your true food preferences. If you struggle to identify your favorite foods, you're not alone. Many people have difficulty identifying which foods satisfy them and in what quantities. In her book *The Diet-Free Revolution*, Alexis Conason (2021) describes diet culture as the loud music that drowns out the internal GPS of true taste preferences. Use the following worksheet to reflect on favorite foods.

Food Enjoyment

How often are you able to enjoy your favorite foods? If you aren't currently eating these foods, how might you be able to begin reincorporating them?

_____

_____

_____

In what ways have life events and diet culture impacted your food choices over your lifetime? _____

_____

_____

_____

Was there ever a time when you remember enjoying food without judgmental thoughts or negative emotions? When—and in what ways—did things shift for you? Recall any messages you received about food or your body that impacted your ability to enjoy food.

_____

_____

_____

Below, we'll give you a tool to assemble everything you've learned in this chapter. First, we will share an example to walk you through this process, and then provide a blank template (also available online) for you to complete.

- *Archer's Story*

  Archer is working on decreasing their binge-eating episodes. They reported the following incident on their self-monitoring forms:

Eating Behavior Exploration, Archer's Example

Day: Saturday

Breakfast: Skipped

Thoughts: I binged again last night. I'm not hungry and feeling discouraged.

Lunch: Burger and fries

Thoughts: I shouldn't eat this food, but it tastes good.

Dinner: Salad with chicken

Thoughts: This is better; I should be eating this more often. I'm still hungry, but I shouldn't be—this is enough food.

Snack: At local ice cream shop, an ice cream sandwich with two cookies and a scoop of ice cream

Thoughts: I don't know the friend who invited me for ice cream very well, and I felt nervous. I asked them not to give me the cookies, but they did. I shouldn't be eating cookies or ice cream. I can't believe I did this.

Other: Binge at home after waking up from a nap after the ice cream: 1 box of Frosted Flakes, ½ bag of Oreos

Thoughts: I still can't believe I ate all that ice cream and cookies. I'm starting over tomorrow but might as well keep eating tonight. I've already screwed today up.

What do you notice about Archer's self-monitoring?

_____

_____

_____

_____

_____

Now that you have made some observations, we will show you how to identify some of the most common triggers for different eating behaviors. Four main categories of triggers can help us understand why certain eating behaviors occur. We'll use Archer's experience as an example.

1. **Dietary Rules:** The experience of following a personal set of eating rules or guidelines can be challenging. Breaking a rule often causes guilt, shame, or embarrassment. Some common responses after breaking a rule might be, "Well, I screwed up again, so I might as well keep eating" or "I can't believe I ate that. I will have to cut back for the rest of the day to make up for this." In Archer's example, does it seem they may feel like they have broken a rule?

   _____

   _____

2. **Undereating:** So far, we have discussed that undereating can include skipping meals or snacks, not having a large enough portion, or not having a variety of foods that feels satisfying. Sometimes, people notice a pattern of undereating in the first part of the day—maybe they are not hungry, saving calories for later, or trying to "make up" for what

they feel was "overeating" or binge eating the night before. In Archer's case, did you identify any undereating on their self-monitoring?

_____

_____

3. **Decreased Awareness:** People often describe experiencing their binge eating or other eating behaviors at times when they are less aware or less focused on what they are doing. There are several reasons this could happen: multitasking, being under the influence of alcohol or other substances, side effects from medication, or feeling overly tired or drowsy. These factors can contribute to a temporary increase in impulsive or distracted behaviors, including eating. For example, if someone is trying to eat their lunch while they are working on an important project, they may not even notice that they have eaten a large bag of potato chips until they stop working. They may also be less aware that they are starting to feel overly full while eating the chips. In Archer's case, do you notice anything that may have caused decreased awareness for them?

_____

_____

4. **Stressful Events or Changes in Mood:** Another common trigger is the occurrence of a stressful event or a change in your mood. This could happen whether the event in question is positive or negative. For example, someone might notice a binge after a stressful day at work. They might notice a similar urge to binge if they are relieved about finishing a large project and want to celebrate. Others might notice changes in their eating behaviors when they are feeling depressed, anxious, lonely, or bored. What do you think about Archer's experience? Do you notice any changes in mood or possible stressful events?

_____

_____

Eating Behavior Exploration

If you have experienced restriction, binge eating, "overeating," "emotional eating," or "undoing" behaviors such as self-induced vomiting, laxative use, or driven exercise, you can use this tool to explore what happened, identify potential triggers, and discover ways to address them in the future.

1. What types of behaviors have you noticed on your self-monitoring forms this week? Select one instance of a behavior you would like to explore.

    _____

    _____

    _____

    _____

2. Describe what happened along with details related to the situation (where you were, who was present, what you were doing).

    _____

    _____

    _____

    _____

3. What types of triggers or contributing factors may have been present for you in this situation? Also use the table below to explore what may be most relevant and what you can change in the future.

    _____

    _____

    _____

    _____

Trigger Category	What You Can Change in the Future

Dietary Rules:
 	
  Thinking about dietary rules or restriction
 	
  Trying to follow dietary rules
 	
  Worrying about breaking a dietary rule
 	
  Feeling guilty after breaking a dietary rule you may have	

Undereating:
 	
  Intentionally skipping meals and/or snacks
 	
  Unintentionally skipping meals and/or snacks
 	
  Going long periods of time in between meals/snacks
 	
  Not eating enough volume of food during the day
 	
  Not eating enough variety of foods during the day	

Decreased Awareness:
 	
  Alcohol use or substance use
 	
  Experiencing side effects from medication
 	
  Feeling tired or drowsy
 	
  Feeling distracted (e.g., watching TV while eating; eating in a social situation)	

Stressful Event or Change in Mood:
 	
  Experiencing a stressful situation or event
 	
  Experiencing negative emotions such as sadness, anger, or anxiety
 	
  Experiencing a positive event or emotions (e.g., feeling relief or wanting to celebrate)	

4.   What patterns have you noticed so far?

_____

_____

5.   What factors contributed to these episodes?

_____

_____

6.   How would you like to address similar situations in the future? Are there other aspects of the situation that may be outside of your control? If so, are there any coping skills that could be helpful to use?

_____

_____

_____

_____

Back to the Hunger Scale Self-Monitoring Form

Now it's time to monitor your hunger on a scale of 1 to 7, with 1 being "too hungry" and 7 being "uncomfortably full." We encourage you to use a new version of the self-monitoring form that has a column to record your hunger and fullness ratings (also available online).

Hunger Scale Self-Monitoring Form

Day/Date: _____

Time	Food Intake	Location	Behavior Restrict (R) Binge (B) Purge (P) Laxatives (L)	Context	Hunger/ Fullness 1 = Too hungry 4 = Neither hungry nor full 7 = Uncomfortably full

Movement:

Summary of Takeaways

Congratulations on finishing chapter 6. Here are some takeaways.

- Increasing the amount and variety of your meals and snacks is key to recovery and may help reduce loss-of-control eating and extreme hunger.

- Incorporating avoided and feared foods regularly is a key strategy to improving your relationship with food.

- Several common factors often maintain disordered eating behaviors: dietary rules, undereating, decreased awareness, and reacting to stressful events and mood changes.

Reflection

What are your takeaways from chapter 6? Take a moment to reflect on anything that surprised you or aspects of the chapter that felt especially relevant to you. What feelings or thoughts came up as you read the information?

_____

_____

_____

_____

_____

When to Move on to Chapter 7

- When you have completed all of the reflection activities in this chapter.

- When you have completed hunger and fullness ratings for at least a week.

- When you have had a chance to use the Eating Behavior Exploration worksheet.

Chapter 7

Making Peace with Your Body

Hello again! In chapter 6, you got ideas for ensuring you are eating enough, gained strategies to help you determine your level of hunger and fullness, and learned how and why it's necessary to break dietary rules. In this chapter, we'll explore body image, weight stigma, and discrimination.

But first we encourage you to complete the following Weekly Progress Tracker (also available online) and then reflect on your experiences with the Hunger-Fullness Scale and the Eating Behavior Exploration worksheet from chapter 6.

Weekly Progress Tracker 3

Take a moment to review your self-monitoring forms from last week and complete the following.

	Day 1	Day 2	Day 3	Day 4	Day 5	Day 6	Day 7
Eating Routines							
Ate breakfast							
Ate lunch							
Ate dinner							
Ate snacks							
Ate every 2–4 hours							
Ate a variety of foods							

	Day 1	Day 2	Day 3	Day 4	Day 5	Day 6	Day 7
Meals kept me feeling satisfied							
Enjoyed the food I was eating							
Other Eating Behaviors							
Restriction							
Binge eating							
Self-induced vomiting							
Laxative use							
Excessive exercise or movement							
Excessive water or caffeine							
Other behaviors (e.g., chewing and spitting, using saunas, etc.)							

What are you noticing about your progress this week?

_____

_____

_____

_____

Now, take a moment to review your Hunger Scale Self-Monitoring Form from last week and complete the following worksheet (also available online) to reflect on the data you collected.

Reflect on Your Hunger Scale Self-Monitoring Form

1	2	3	4	5	6	7
Too hungry		Neither hungry nor full			So uncomfortably full	

Did you find you were hungry (below a 3) before meals?

_____

Did you find you were full (above a 5) after meals?

_____

Were there times you let your hunger get extreme (below a 2)? What happened?

_____

Were there times you ate beyond fullness (to 6 or above)? What did you notice?

_____

_____

What changes to your eating plan do you want to make this week? For example, should the size of one of your meals or snacks be modified? Or should the timing of meals change? It's also okay if you don't have a specific goal in mind. Maybe you just want to continue exploring emotions and behaviors.

_____

_____

What Is Body Image?

When you read the term "body image," what comes to mind? Take a moment to write down what this concept means to you.

_____

_____

_____

_____

_____

Body image is multidimensional and complex (Cash 2008). It is also related to cultural beliefs, ableism, fatphobia, capitalism, and patriarchy. It includes physical sensations, thoughts, and emotions about your body. Behaviors displayed toward our bodies—including positive acts of self-care—are also influenced by and impact our body image. Sunscreen applications, safe sex practices, and honoring your body's need for rest are just a few examples. Body image spans beyond weight and shape to include aspects of our appearance, such as the shape and size of our facial features and body parts, physical disabilities, hair texture, and skin color, among other details. The degree to which our physical appearance aligns with our gender identity is another important piece of the body image puzzle. Our cultural identities may also shape beliefs about our physical traits.

When you wrote out your definition of body image, did it include more than just the size and shape of your body? What other traits did you include?

_____

_____

_____

When you are asked to picture an "attractive" body, what characteristics (or physical traits) come to mind? What impact do you believe the media and unique aspects of your culture have had in defining these characteristics?

_____

_____

_____

_____

Negative Body Image and Its Impact

Unfortunately, in American society, dissatisfaction with our bodies is the norm. Known as "normative discontent," this concept is present among many people who do not have eating disorders (Rodin, Silberstein, and Moore 1984; Tantleff-Dunn, Barnes, and Larose 2011). How a person reacts in response to that discontent varies. Sometimes, it can start as an innocent attempt to feel better in one's body or to "get healthier."

People aren't always aware of the large amount of "mental real estate" that food, weight, and shape concerns occupy in their brains. You might find that your thoughts about your body shape and weight take up much mental time and energy. This can make it hard to show up in other areas of life, such as work, school, parenting, friendships, or leisure activities. Perhaps you show up physically in life but notice that you're mentally absent and disengaged. Like a smartphone on low battery with unused apps open in the background, your eating disorder can continually sap your energy. Review the following image of the brain and then think about the past week.

Compare to my friends

Hobbies

Is this healthy?

Scale

Calories

Work

Weight

Protein

Avoid

Clothes feel tight

My dog

Friends

Current events

Family

Social media

Exercise

Control

Check my Body

Walk

Survive life

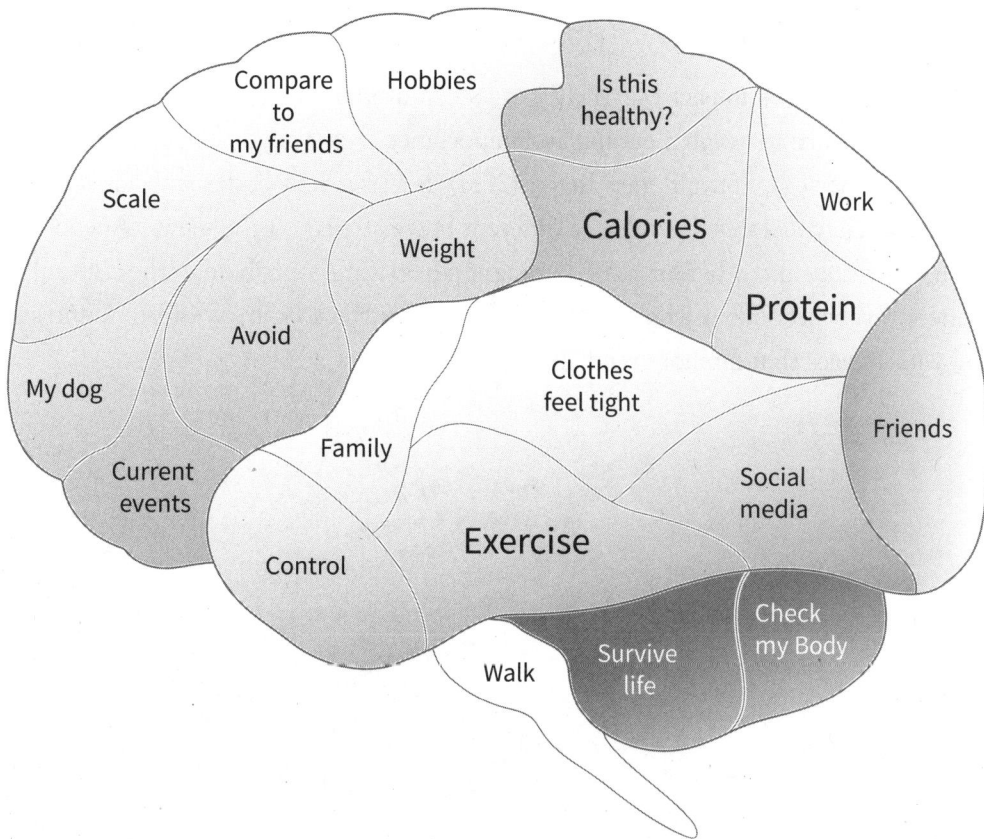

What would a representation of your brain energy look like?

_____

_____

_____

With which areas of life does your concern about your body interfere?

_____

_____

_____

Body Image Influences

Several different factors impact our body image. On a broad level, societal and political influences affect how we learn to assign meaning and importance to our physical appearance. In her book *The Body Is Not an Apology*, Sonya Renee Taylor (2021) describes how bodies are classified in a "hierarchy" in which society dictates the value of different bodies based on the views of people in power. Social media, television, and other forms of dominant advertising contribute to the cultural narrative that influences our beliefs about what is attractive and unattractive. In Western countries, we are bombarded with images that promote rigid appearance ideals.

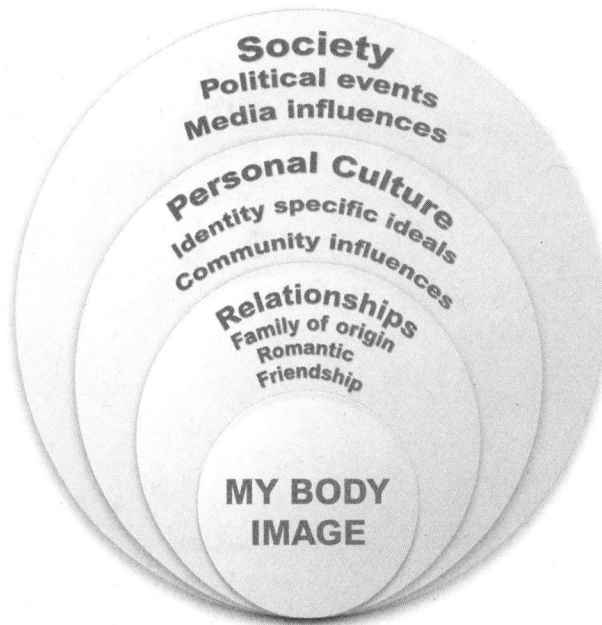

Society
Political events
Media influences

Personal Culture
Identity specific ideals
Community influences

Relationships
Family of origin
Romantic
Friendship

MY BODY IMAGE

Take a moment to reflect on societal and political influences on your views of your body. Examples include the television programs you watched as a child, magazines you read as a teen, or social media influencers you follow as an adult.

_____

_____

_____

Your cultural and community appearance ideals can also influence your body image. For example, certain cultures may view larger bodies as more prosperous and attractive than smaller bodies. Other communities, such as gym subcultures, may value large muscles over a thin appearance. Religious communities may uphold certain expectations about the visibility of specific body parts that influence how people view their bodies. Your social community might place a high value on fitting in and look down on appearances that seem different from what is considered "normal."

> Record any relevant cultural and community influences on your body image. Remember that these influences may be positive, neutral, or negative. For example, people who practice religious modesty may have some protection from cultural body image ideals. Other examples might include your geographic region's emphasis on fitness or appearance ideals within your work setting.
>
> _____
>
> _____
>
> _____

Finally, interpersonal experiences with others impact how we view our bodies. The feedback we receive from important others is shown to be the most influential in developing attitudes toward our bodies (Lawrence et al. 2022; Lawrence et al. 2023). Consider the positive influence that a parent or teacher can have when they model appreciation of body diversity and refrain from making disparaging comments about their bodies. On the flip side, peers who tease or discriminate based on the color or texture of one's skin, hair type, or body shape and size can leave lasting scars.

> Write some examples of interpersonal experiences that have impacted your body image.
>
> _____
>
> _____
>
> _____
>
> _____
>
> _____

Everybody—and every body—has a history. The more years we live, the more our narrative expands. The world treats bodies differently, but that doesn't have to determine how we treat or feel about our bodies.

Using a blank piece of paper, create a body timeline. Consider including influential events and activities, relationships, or societal messages that may have impacted your views of your body and appearance over the years as points on your timeline. Remember to consider both negative *and* positive influences. You could also record the status of your eating disorder behaviors over time.

Once you have completed your timeline, use the following worksheet to reflect on what you have included.

Exploring Your Body Timeline

How have the different points on your timeline influenced your beliefs about bodies *in general*?

_____

_____

_____

How have points on your timeline influenced the beliefs or expectations for *your own body*? Are they the same as what you described above? If you hold different expectations for your body, why might this be?

_____

_____

_____

_____

_____

When you think about these beliefs, what emotions do you experience? What behaviors are you compelled to do (or not do)?

_____

_____

_____

_____

_____

_____

As an example of a body narrative, below is an excerpt from Virgie Tovar's 2018 book *You Have the Right to Remain Fat*. Virgie is an author and leading expert in weight-based discrimination. In this excerpt, Virgie describes an early memory of being in her body:

"When I was a little girl...when we got home from errands or preschool...I would take all my clothes off as quickly as possible...I would leave the pile on the floor and then run back out, giggle with uncontained delight, to the kitchen where my grandmother was always cooking...

I would spread out my arms and legs as far as I could. And I would jiggle. My thighs and belly, my cheeks and my whole body would wobble. I would turn my head in circles. I liked that everything moved and undulated. My body was like the water in the bathtub or the water at the community pool, which I loved so much in the summer. My body was like that water, a source of relief and fun, a place I could jump into and be held. It felt good..."

What reactions do you notice after reading this?

_____

_____

How are you doing after reflecting on these body image topics and creating your timeline? We recognize that these activities can bring up many complex emotions and thoughts. We invite you to take a moment to take a breath and acknowledge any difficulty you've faced in your body over the years. Offer yourself kindness and compassion—consider reviewing the self-compassion information in chapter 5—then return to the present and look forward.

Weight Stigma, Bias, and Discrimination

What is weight stigma, and how do we internalize it in the first place? Weight stigma is defined as the discrimination or stereotyping of people based on their weight or body size. A related term, weight bias, describes the negative attitudes and beliefs about people due to their weight. While the experience of weight stigma is most common among people with larger bodies, it can be experienced by people of any size. However, the consequences of weight stigma are much worse for those in larger bodies and for those experiencing other intersecting forms of oppression.

As explained in Sabrina Strings's 2019 book, *Fearing the Black Body: The Racial Origins of Fat Phobia*, weight stigma and bias are rooted in both racism and sexism and are tied to the presence of the transatlantic slave trade in the United States. Colonizers often viewed fatness as a sign of immorality and racial inferiority, and Black people were frequently portrayed as being in larger bodies due to gluttony and love of food. Women, and especially Black women, have also experienced more weight stigma than men across the centuries due in large part to the emphasis on thinness in beauty standards in North American culture. As we noted in chapter 2, the BMI also has origins rooted in racism and sexism. Unfortunately, the BMI is still commonly used by most health care providers and often serves as gatekeeping for many interventions, including certain medications, orthopedic surgeries, and gender-affirming care.

Most of us are exposed to weight stigma and bias from an early age, including media, social media, friends, family, and even health care professionals. One study found that health care providers are the second most common source of weight stigma and that over 53 percent of people with larger bodies have experienced inappropriate comments from their doctor about their weight (Puhl, Andreyeva, and Brownell 2008). Weight stigma is so pervasive that it even appears in children's television shows (Eisenberg et al. 2014). Many people who are exposed to weight stigma and bias may also internalize these experiences. So, what do weight stigma and bias look like? Here are some common examples:

- Lack of access to eating disorder care

- Ridicule, name-calling, or negative or derogatory comments about weight or body size

- Unsolicited comments about body size and advice or compliments about weight loss

- Lack of comfortable seating in the workplace, restaurants, public transportation, stores, and airplanes

- Lack of appropriate seating, gowns, and/or medical equipment (e.g., exam tables, blood pressure cuff, immunization syringes, scales) at a health care provider's office

- Limited access to clothing that you would like to purchase in your size in a store, or only being able to shop online

- Denial of medical treatment due to weight or being told that weight loss is required to receive a certain treatment

- Fewer promotions, lower pay, and harsher disciplinary actions in workplace settings

- Lack of representation of people in larger bodies in television, movies, theater, and the music industry

Weight stigma and bias can cause negative effects in several different areas. People who have encountered weight stigma are more likely to experience body dissatisfaction, greater psychological distress, more frequent disordered eating behaviors, and poorer quality of life (Levinson et al. 2023). Weight stigma is also a risk factor for physical issues such as increased inflammation, high blood pressure, and higher blood sugar levels (Puhl and Suh 2015; Tomiyama et al. 2018). When people experience weight stigma and bias, they are also less likely to seek health care, which can lead to delays in diagnosis and treatment. Often, when people finally do seek treatment, their weight is blamed for any health concerns, which worsens the experience of this stigma.

How do you know whether you have internalized weight stigma and bias? The following are some signs to consider. Check any that apply.

- ☐ Avoiding having your picture taken

- ☐ Avoiding mirrors or reflections

- ☐ Criticizing your weight and/or body size

- ☐ Avoiding social situations due to concerns about weight

- ☐ Avoiding being naked or intimate with a partner

- ☐ Avoiding wearing certain types of clothing (e.g., sleeveless shirts, shorts, or form-fitting clothes)

☐ Avoiding health care due to fear of comments about your weight

☐ Fear or anxiety related to eating in front of others

☐ Engaging in frequent dieting, exercise, or other strategies to change weight or body size

☐ Avoiding sports, gyms, or other physical activity due to fear of judgment

☐ Holding off on job changes, dating, or other opportunities in your life until you reach your "goal weight"

If you have a smaller body size, you may be thinking, "Can I really experience internalized weight bias?" The answer is *yes*. Even observing the negative treatment of others due to their weight and body size can lead to internalized weight bias. This can contribute to fears associated with weight gain and increased behaviors to control or maintain weight. The following worksheet will help you think about your experience with weight bias.

Internalized Weight Bias

What did you learn about people in larger bodies growing up in your family and with your peers? How was weight and body size discussed? How did family members address changes in people's body size?

_____

_____

What were you exposed to regarding weight/body size on television, movies, and other media you watched growing up? What kinds of patterns did you notice about people in larger bodies in the media?

_____

_____

What has your experience been in the health care system? How has your weight been discussed? How have you been treated when there have been changes in your weight?

_____

_____

Have you experienced or witnessed any of the other examples of weight bias described above? What were those experiences like for you?

_____

_____

How have other aspects of your identity intersected with experiences of weight bias? For example, how has your race, gender, or sexual orientation played a role in how your weight and or body size has been perceived?

_____

_____

Unlearning Internalized Weight Bias

Now that you have had a chance to reflect on your experiences with weight stigma, bias, and discrimination, it's time to start unlearning. Some of the strategies that can help shift beliefs in these areas include:

- Increase awareness of the impact of weight stigma and diet culture and how it shows up in your day-to-day life. Look at some books, articles, and podcasts related to this topic that we have included in the online resources.

- Reflect on how you have been impacted by weight stigma and bias in your life. Consider journaling, talking with friends, or exploring this with your therapist.

- Clean up your social media feed. Consider removing or reducing sources that seem to be rooted in diet culture and weight stigma.

- Diversify your social media feed with sources highlighting non-diet approaches, body neutrality, body diversity, body acceptance, and fat liberation content. Try to follow people of various bodies, including people of different sizes, abilities, genders, races, and ethnicities.

- Seek a community of others who want to reduce weight stigma and bias. See chapter 9 for more guidance in this area!

- Find weight-inclusive health care providers that make you feel comfortable seeking care (see chapter 1).

- Find ways to care for your body at any size. In the online resources, see our Caring for Fat Bodies guide.

As you start to learn more about the process of unlearning weight bias, you might consider reclaiming the word "fat" as a neutral descriptor. For many people addressing internalized weight bias, this can be helpful. If you live in a larger body, you may not feel ready to describe yourself as "fat"—and that is okay too! In the following worksheet, we invite you to reflect on what this word means to you and what it might feel like to use the word to describe your body.

Reclaiming the Word "Fat" and Fat Positivity

What does the word "fat" mean to you?

_____

_____

What thoughts, feelings, and physical sensations appear when you hear the word "fat"? How about using it to describe yourself?

_____

_____

How would it feel to start using the word "fat" to describe yourself if you are living in a larger body? How would it feel if a friend or family member started reclaiming this term for themselves?

_____

_____

We want to stress that there is no pressure to use this term as part of your journey to unlearn weight bias. Many people prefer using the terms "larger body," "bigger," or "higher weight" (Robbins et al. 2025). We do recommend avoiding the terms "overweight" and "obese," as these terms are linked to the BMI, which, as previously noted, is rooted in weight bias, racism, and sexism.

Body Checking and Avoidance

Given the pervasiveness of weight bias, we cannot entirely escape it. These next strategies will focus on what you can change. These two categories of behaviors are called *body checking* and *body avoidance*.

Body Checking and Comparing

Body-checking behaviors are repetitive behaviors that typically involve analyzing or judging different aspects of your body. This can include behaviors such as:

- Frequent weighing

- Mirror or reflection checking

- Examining photos or scrutinizing selfies

- Checking clothing fit

- Checking your body by pinching or touching different areas

- Measuring parts of your body

- Checking to see how your body compares to those around you

- Asking for feedback on appearance

- Comparing yourself to past photos

Of course, it is typical to have some level of checking behaviors. For example, most people glance in the mirror before leaving the house to check their appearance. This type of behavior is typically brief, does not interfere with other activities, and does not cause a significant amount of distress that can continue throughout the day. Unhelpful body checking tends to be repetitive, takes up long periods of time, interferes with other activities, causes people to be late, incurs significant emotional distress, and can often encourage ongoing negative thoughts or urges to keep checking. It can also lead to the use of eating disorder behaviors.

The following figure demonstrates a common cycle that occurs with body checking. It can provide temporary relief, but anxiety about appearance can quickly build up again. This cycle is hard to break without reducing the checking behaviors themselves. Use the following worksheet to explore your own body-checking behaviors.

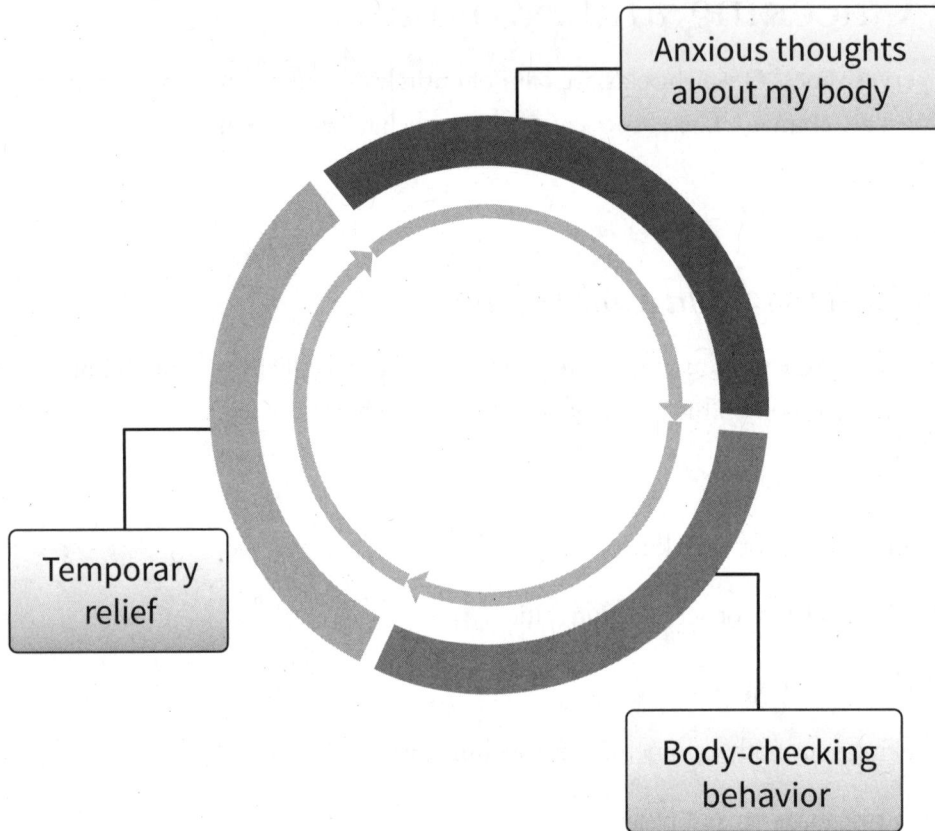

Body-Checking Behaviors

Which checking behaviors have you noticed yourself using?

_____

_____

How much time are you spending on these behaviors? Do they interfere with other things you would like to do?

_____

_____

Why do you think you spend time on these behaviors? Do they seem helpful in some way?

_____

_____

How do you feel during and after these checking behaviors? What thoughts do you notice about yourself and your body? What emotions do you experience?

_____

_____

If comparing yourself to others, to whom do you tend to compare yourself? Is it people you see day to day in real life or on social media? How does it make you feel? Is it helpful?

_____

_____

Based on these reflection questions, are there any checking or comparing behaviors that you might want to reduce?

_____

_____

If you have identified some behaviors you would like to reduce, consider using the following strategies. We recommend starting with just one or two behaviors at a time to make the process feel less overwhelming.

- Consider time limits for checking behaviors, such as limiting the duration of your mirror checks to under five minutes.

- Consider limiting certain checking behaviors by the number of times per day or week. For example, many people find it helpful to limit or eliminate how often they check the scale. You can either gradually decrease your number of checks or enforce a maximum limit immediately.

- If it's hard to limit the time spent on certain checking behaviors, consider making aspects less accessible. For example, covering or removing mirrors around the house can help reduce mirror-checking behavior. Or you could wear clothing that makes body checking harder.

- If you notice an urge to pinch or check your body, substitute a compassionate touch, such as a self-hug or brief self-massage.

- Instead of comparing your body to others, think about something you appreciate or admire about that other person.

- If this feels overwhelming to do yourself, ask a support person for help. For example, some people find it helpful to ask a family member or friend to assist them by removing things such as scales and mirrors that may be involved in body checking.

- If you ask for feedback or reassurance from others about your appearance, consider letting others know that you are trying to change this behavior so that they can support you in making this change.

- Have some enjoyable, distracting activities ready when you resist the urge to check. This could be a new book, a favorite TV show, spending time with your pet, or calling a supportive friend.

- Consider decorating mirrors and reflective surfaces with body-positive messages.

- When you notice urges to check, set a timer and try sitting with the urge for increasing amounts of time.

Body Avoidance

Body avoidance is the second category of behaviors that can maintain body image concerns. Even though this behavior may seem like the opposite of body checking, people commonly engage in a complex mix of these behaviors. Body-avoidance behaviors typically include strategies to avoid looking at your body and strategies to prevent other people from seeing your body. Avoidance behaviors related to seeing your body could include avoiding mirrors or reflections, shopping for clothing, self-care activities that involve touching the body—such as applying lotion or sunscreen—or looking at photographs of yourself. Avoidance behaviors related to others seeing your body might include avoiding wearing certain types of clothing; wearing swimwear at the pool or the beach; close physical contact with others, such as hugging or sexual intimacy; and photographs or videos. As illustrated in the following figure, body-avoidance behaviors are related to fears of negative outcomes. Avoidance can provide temporary relief but maintain the fear associated with these situations.

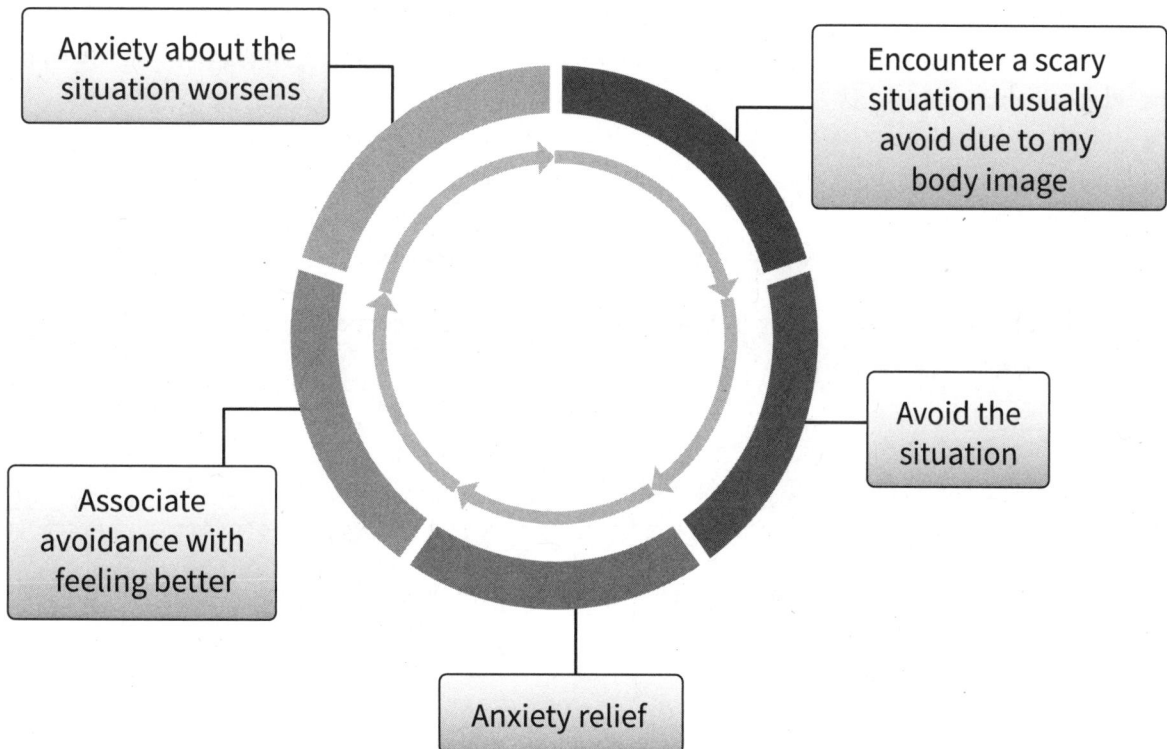

Exposure is usually recommended to challenge the expected outcome. However, this can be unhelpful and invalidating for people in larger bodies, or with other marginalized identities, who may have valid fears regarding certain situations. For example, if you are in a larger body and avoid looking in the mirror to prevent negative emotions, this might be related to internalized weight bias from years of negative treatment from peers, family members, and health care providers. Exposure to your reflection is not going to convince you that your body is not large. Validation of your experience may be more helpful. Similarly, if you have avoided shopping due to fears of being unable to find clothing in your size, sending you on a shopping trip to a store that lacks inclusive sizing might reinforce these fears. Or, if you have avoided eating certain foods in front of others and go out to eat, you may receive unwanted comments about your food choices.

We acknowledge the possibility of negative experiences with exposure. We can't fully control how the world responds, and you may encounter bias (Pinciotti et al. 2022). However, challenging yourself to explore behaviors you have avoided and building tolerance to what comes has been shown to help many people lead more fulfilling lives (Kesby et al. 2017). We invite you to think about which avoided behaviors are most important to you and might be meaningful to add back into your life (Butler and Levinson 2024). For example, if going out to eat with friends fits in with your value of building relationships with others, it may be helpful to push through the discomfort of potential negative outcomes to have that experience. Use the following worksheet to explore your own body-avoidance behaviors.

Body-Avoidance Behaviors

Have you noticed yourself engaging in any of the avoidance behaviors discussed earlier? If so, which ones can you relate to the most?

_____

_____

Consider the behaviors you're avoiding. How might avoidance be protecting you? Reflect on the pros and cons of your avoidance behaviors.

_____

_____

Given these pros and cons, would the benefits of facing this situation outweigh the potential cons? Would this involve being in a situation that would make you feel unsafe? If yes, are there alternatives that you could start with instead?

_____

_____

What would it be like to challenge yourself to engage in some of these avoided behaviors? Are there any potential benefits to adding these behaviors back into your life?

_____

_____

What is one behavior or activity that you might be open to exploring? What would it look like to gradually add this back in?

_____

_____

When you think about adding this behavior or activity back in, what causes you anxiety?

_____

_____

Are there supportive people who could help you change your avoidance behaviors?

_____

_____

If you have identified some behaviors you would like to change, consider using the following strategies. We recommend starting with just one or two behaviors at a time to make the process feel less overwhelming.

- Bring awareness to your thoughts, feelings, or physical sensations while attempting to engage in the avoided behavior. Don't try to challenge or change these reactions—they are your valid responses to a challenging situation. Try to sit with these responses and remind yourself that with time and continued practice, the intensity will decrease.

- Consider how your reactions tie into past experiences with these avoided behaviors. Acknowledge that these are natural reactions if these behaviors have led to negative experiences in the past.

- Focus on any positive aspects of the experience. Is this something that you might enjoy more if you can do this again in the future? Will this add anything to your life?

- ## *Jeff's Story*

Jeff is a forty-five-year-old man. He experienced a lot of teasing from his peers and family members during childhood because of his body size, and he worked hard to lose weight to join the Army after graduating from high school. Jeff had difficulty maintaining his new weight in the military, especially after basic training ended. He started to learn purging strategies from his peers that seemed to help him lose weight quickly and "make weight" during PT tests. After his discharge from the Army Jeff noticed that his weight continued to increase over time. He avoided eating out with friends due to shame and fears of being judged for his eating. He missed the social interaction but felt increasingly uncomfortable with the idea of eating around other people.

Jeff and his therapist started to identify body-checking and body-avoidance behaviors to change. Since social engagement was an important value to Jeff, he decided to challenge himself to start going out to lunch with his friends again. Initially, the experience was challenging. Jeff had difficulty fitting into the booth at the restaurant his friends had chosen, and he noticed that his friends spent a lot of time commenting on each other's food choices. However, Jeff decided to try again because he really enjoyed catching up with his friends.

Jeff's therapist encouraged him to check out fat acceptance social media accounts run by men and other body-positive media showing fat people living joyously. Over time, Jeff started to feel more comfortable. He could tune out the comments about food choices, started advocating for restaurants with more comfortable seating, and even shared some of the information he learned about weight bias with his friends.

Addressing Body Changes

If you have gained weight or are gaining weight throughout recovery, the body changes you experience can feel cruel. Facing your core fear directly can be intensely dysregulating. This is understandable, especially if you are living in a larger body or growing into one. You have absorbed cultural messages that fatness and weight gain are bad. Hopefully, by now, you're questioning this perspective and coming to a more accepting position. However, changes like these take time.

It's also easy to romanticize a time in your life when your body was smaller. But if you have spent time at a lower weight, you may have struggled when you were at that weight. Now might be a good time to revisit why you picked up this book—review your advantages and challenges list from chapter 1.

• *Claudia's Story*

Claudia remembers how good it felt to be thin, when she could wear her favorite clothes, shop in any store, and attract looks as she walked into a bar. She longs to go back to that body. Claudia romanticizes a time when she was thinner.

Her friend questioned whether that time was really so great. Claudia, when pushed, remembers that she was so afraid she'd be tempted to eat that she couldn't really go out on dates. She was often depressed and irritable. Her life, in fact, was very small.

Use the following worksheet to explore your feelings about body changes.

Exploring Body Changes

How might body changes objectively impact you? For example, would you need to buy new clothes? Shop elsewhere? Would it affect your relationships? Your ability to have relationships? Your ability to find work?

_____

_____

_____

_____

We don't want to sugarcoat it. Such body changes are challenging, and it's normal to feel scared. But what is the cost of fighting your body's set point?

_____

_____

Having a body is a guarantee of uncertainty because it changes over time. Have there been other times in your life when you've tolerated change? Could you use similar strategies to help you now?

_____

_____

If you long for a time in your life when you were thinner, ask yourself: Were there negative consequences of dieting and weight suppression that you tend to sugarcoat in retrospect?

_____

_____

What are some potential advantages—such as less food obsession and fewer binge episodes—of being at a higher weight?

_____

_____

Is it possible that it won't be as bad as you fear? Think about another time when you were afraid and consider whether the outcome was as bad as you feared. Many people imagine their worst-case scenario, and most often, reality is not as bad as they feared.

_____

_____

Sizing Up

During your recovery process, you may find that at some point, your clothes no longer fit. This can be very distressing; our culture sends many disordered messages that this is a bad thing. You may find women who brag online about still fitting into their high school jeans. But remember what we told you about bodies continuing to add mass through adulthood.

We have found that people of any size who gain weight in recovery often experience a sense of failure when their clothing size increases. This is no surprise: Our culture overvalues thinness. But continuing to wear undersized clothing is uncomfortable physically and mentally. And continuing to look at clothes that don't fit you only increases distress. Buying bigger clothing is often necessary.

We find that for many people, the dread over having to replace the clothing—and in the meantime, having to face the clothing that doesn't fit—is the hardest part. But once they have clothes that fit well and feel more comfortable physically, they feel more able to face the world, and getting dressed each morning is no longer an occasion for self-deprecation.

Bodies age and change in ways that we can't control. We need to accept that. If finances allow, our advice is always to buy a few basic things that fit you well and help you to feel great and put the other clothes out of sight for now. If you are in a larger body, we know it can be challenging to find clothing that fits, especially in stores. We have provided some online resources that may help. No matter what your eating disorder tells you, you deserve to have clothes that fit you.

What barriers are preventing you from wearing more comfortable clothing? Here are some common concerns and follow-up ideas to consider:

- "I don't want to wear a larger size; I'm having trouble letting go of clothing in smaller sizes."

    What does your clothing tag size say about you as a person?

    _____

- "I have positive memories in those clothes."

    If you find yourself hesitant to let go of clothing pieces from a certain time, are there ways to remake them to fit your current life? For example, would those dresses make a quilt, or can those jeans be remade into a skirt or jacket? Can you give them to your niece or a friend's daughter who can make new memories in those bell-bottom jeans that are now back in style again?

_____

_____

_____

- "I can't afford new clothes."

  This can be challenging, especially when trying to access larger clothing sizes at fair prices. One idea is to search online for community clothing swaps near you. Check out the resources section for more ideas.

Grieving

As part of this process, you may finally abandon the hope of attaining or returning to a thinner body. This may have been a significant focus for your time and energy for many years. You may have spent years dieting and trying to get your body smaller and postponed activities such as travel, dating, and shopping until you'd achieved that ideal body. Grieving can be a natural part of the recovery process, and it often helps to lean into the experience to keep moving forward. The following worksheet may help you explore this.

Grieving Your Ideal Body

What does it feel like to give up on that dream for your ideal body? You may feel upset about wasted time, loss of dreams, and fear, among other things. Anything else?

_____

_____

_____

What does it feel like to accept your body as it is now? What feelings does that evoke?

_____

_____

_____

If you accept your body's higher weight, that may mean giving up the hope of participating in certain activities such as horseback riding, ziplining, and amusement park rides that have weight restrictions. Write about grieving these potential activities.

_____

_____

_____

_____

What other activities can you do? How might your life be more fulfilling without the eating disorder?

_____

_____

_____

You may also feel sad about giving up your eating disorder, which has seen you through some tough times and helped you cope. Letting go can create feelings of sadness. How do you feel about giving up your eating disorder?

_____

_____

_____

Finally, you may never stop wanting to lose weight. But what would it be like to accept that and move on?

_____

_____

_____

Episodes of Body Discomfort

Regardless of body size, you may experience episodes of discomfort in your body. These negative body image episodes may be either chronic or acute. Acute episodes can be triggered by seeing yourself in a reflection or photo, comparing yourself to others, or other situations such as rejection. They may be accompanied by shame, sadness, frustration, or other negative emotions. These experiences can worsen negative body image and low self-esteem and maintain eating problems (Srivastava et al. 2024). The following worksheet (also available online) may help you explore this.

Exploring Episodes of Body Discomfort

Some people with eating and body issues tend to project many—if not all—negative emotions onto their bodies. For example, think about the last time you felt negatively about your body. When was it?

_____

_____

_____

What happened just before you felt bad in your body? Did you experience any triggers? What were they?

_____

_____

_____

Did you experience feelings such as guilt, disgust, sadness, frustration, boredom? Did you feel unworthy, unlovable, or inferior? What feelings came up for you?

_____

_____

_____

You may be aware of sensations, such as feeling clothes on your body, body parts touching, heat or sweatiness, and more. What sensations did you feel in your body?

_____

_____

_____

When you experience a negative emotion or uncomfortable sensation, do you project it onto your body or blame your body?

_____

_____

_____

Look back at your symptom map from chapter 2 and see whether you can connect episodes of feeling bad in your body to other eating behaviors.

_____

_____

_____

_____

The next time you experience an intense episode of negative body image, take yourself through the previous exercise. Try to identify at least one underlying feeling. You can look at the Feelings Wheel in the online resources. Try just to tolerate the feelings that arise without using an eating disorder behavior. Or use the coping skills from chapter 5. Then, show your body some appreciation.

Body Appreciation

Body appreciation is accepting, holding positive attitudes toward, and respecting the body (Tylka and Wood-Barcalow 2015a). It involves praising the body for what it can do, what it represents, and its diverse features (Tylka and Wood-Barcalow 2015b). People with higher levels of body appreciation have been shown to feel better about themselves and have better sexual satisfaction—as well as lower levels of disordered eating (Linardon et al. 2022).

- *Ezra's Story*

  Ezra has been struggling with eating disorder symptoms for many years. Still, as a person living with multiple chronic illnesses and disabilities, they have often felt like these symptoms are overlooked or dismissed by their providers. When they were finally able to seek treatment, they had a difficult time connecting with the content related to improving body image concerns. As a person with disabilities, Ezra has found it challenging to balance appearance ideals in terms of weight, shape, and ability. When considering body appreciation, Ezra often focuses on what their body cannot do currently.

  Ezra decides to take a different approach by seeking out community through social media and local disability activism groups. Self-expression through clothing, hair, and accessories helps them feel more empowered about their appearance. They start to appreciate the abilities they do have and the diversity of abilities in the community they have joined. They create a list of positive qualities about themselves that do not focus only on physical attributes and find that this helps improve their sense of self-worth. They also take steps to spend more time on self-care and permit themselves to rest, take breaks, and set boundaries when needed.

Does any aspect of Ezra's story resonate with you? In what ways can you appreciate your body? Consider what tasks your body helps you complete and how it can provide pleasure.

_____

_____

_____

_____

_____

Rethinking Your Relationship with Movement

One major aspect of diet culture is the focus on exercise and physical activity for the purposes of weight loss and changing your body shape or size. As you let go of weight bias and build an appreciation for your body, you might want to rebuild your relationship with movement (however, if certain types of physical activity have been a part of your eating disorder in the past, we recommend reintroducing these activities with caution). Use the following worksheet (also available online) to explore your experiences with movement in the past and how it might look for you in the future. You might also revisit the online resource Addressing Excessive Exercise.

What was your experience with physical activity and exercise during childhood? Did you enjoy any sports, dance, or other movement-related activities? Did you feel pressured to take part in any activities?

_____

_____

What types of physical movement or activity have you enjoyed as an adult? What has felt fun for you?

_____

_____

How do you feel when you think about engaging in physical movement or activity now? What reactions do you have?

_____

_____

Are there any activities that you would like to explore? What might hold you back from trying out these new activities?

_____

_____

Are there activities that you can enjoy with others?

_____

_____

• _Susan's Story_

Susan is a twenty-five-year-old woman who was a multi-sport athlete throughout middle school and high school. As a child, she was larger than her peers and often encouraged to lose weight by her pediatrician. When she first started playing soccer in elementary school, she lost weight and received praise from her parents and other relatives for the changes in her body. Susan loved soccer and enjoyed playing it, and she had not even noticed the connection between this new sport and the changes in her body until it was pointed out to her.

As Susan continued through middle and high school, she became more and more concerned about keeping up "enough" activity to maintain her weight loss. She still enjoyed soccer, but felt pressured to complete extra workouts outside of practice to ensure she was burning enough calories. She started to experience fatigue and energy loss, and her performance on the field began to suffer. Susan also noticed fluctuations in her weight, and she began restricting her food intake more to try to avoid any weight gain. By the time she graduated from high school, she was relieved to have finished with soccer.

Years later, Susan continues to struggle with restrictive eating. She avoids physical activity due to her prior focus on exercise to burn calories, lose weight, and maintain a certain body size. As Susan starts to address her disordered eating behaviors, she considers what type of physical activity might be enjoyable for her. Susan realizes that she misses the sense of teamwork that she loved so much when she first started playing soccer. She learns about a kickball team from a coworker and decides to try it out after work one day. Susan has a great time and realizes that this might be a fun way to incorporate some movement into her weekly routine that also involves socializing.

Susan also learns to tune in to how her body feels and how to respond compassionately. She has noticed some stiffness in her muscles and joints at the end of the day and has decided to try some gentle stretching a few days a week. She finds an online, weight-inclusive yoga instructor and starts taking classes that allow her to feel safe and supported in this new type of movement.

Susan is sometimes tempted to engage in other activities, such as running, to burn more calories again. She recognizes that this is the only reason she wants to consider running. She decides to continue engaging in the fun movement, which feels good physically and seems easy to maintain.

Some of the most powerful body image–related interventions come from individuals with lived experience in marginalized bodies. We include these in our online resources. We also strongly recommend the comprehensive resource *Positive Body Image Workbook* (Wood-Barcalow, Tylka, and Judge 2021).

Summary of Takeaways

Congratulations on finishing chapter 7! In this chapter, we explored:

- The multiple influences of body image from your personal relationships, community, and society.

- How body checking and avoidance can maintain your eating disorder.

- Ways to start unlearning weight bias.

- The powerful role that body appreciation and acceptance play in reducing body image distress.

Reflection

What are your takeaways from chapter 7? Take a moment to reflect on anything that surprised you and aspects of the chapter that were relevant to you. What feelings or thoughts arose as you read the information?

_____

_____

_____

_____

_____

_____

When to Move on to Chapter 8

- You've completed all relevant reflection activities in this chapter.

- You feel ready to delve deeper into self-esteem.

Chapter 8

Self-Esteem, Thoughts, Beliefs, and Perfectionism

When you think about self-esteem, what comes to mind? What parts of your identity contribute to how you feel about yourself overall? Many who have struggled with their eating and body image may find that thoughts about their body weight, shape, and appearance play a large role in terms of self-esteem. The following activities are designed to broaden your sense of self-worth. First, let's check in with how things have been going with the Weekly Progress Tracker (also available online). As with every new chapter, take a few moments to review your self-monitoring forms from the last week.

Weekly Progress Tracker 4

	Day 1	Day 2	Day 3	Day 4	Day 5	Day 6	Day 7
Eating Routines							
Ate breakfast							
Ate lunch							
Ate dinner							
Ate snacks							
Ate every 2–4 hours							

	Day 1	Day 2	Day 3	Day 4	Day 5	Day 6	Day 7
Ate a variety of foods							
Meals kept me feeling satisfied							
Enjoyed the food I was eating							
Other Eating Behaviors							
Restriction							
Binge eating							
Self-induced vomiting							
Laxative use							
Excessive exercise or movement							
Excessive water or caffeine							
Body checking							
Body avoidance							
Other behaviors (e.g., chewing and spitting, using saunas, etc.)							

What are you noticing about your progress this week?

_____

_____

_____

Allocation of Time, Energy, and Resources on Weight Concerns

You may recall that earlier in the workbook, we asked you to consider the mental real estate that weight and shape concerns may occupy in your mind. The following pie chart activity is a similar exercise that asks you to consider how you allocate your time, energy, and resources across different areas of your life. How would you like this to shift in the future? Below, we share an example from Maria, and then provide a worksheet (also available online) for you to complete.

- *Maria's Story*

  When Maria first sat down to complete the pie chart activity, she felt ashamed to consider the time and energy she had spent on her weight and shape concerns. She considered how much time she spent checking her weight or looking in the mirror, researching diets online, looking at weight loss success stories on social media, and comparing herself to past pictures. She realized that she had probably spent at least 50 percent of her spare time doing something or thinking about something related to her worries about her weight, shape, and how she looked. As a result, she also noticed that she had less time for hobbies that she enjoyed and less time for her friends.

Maria's Pie Chart Currently

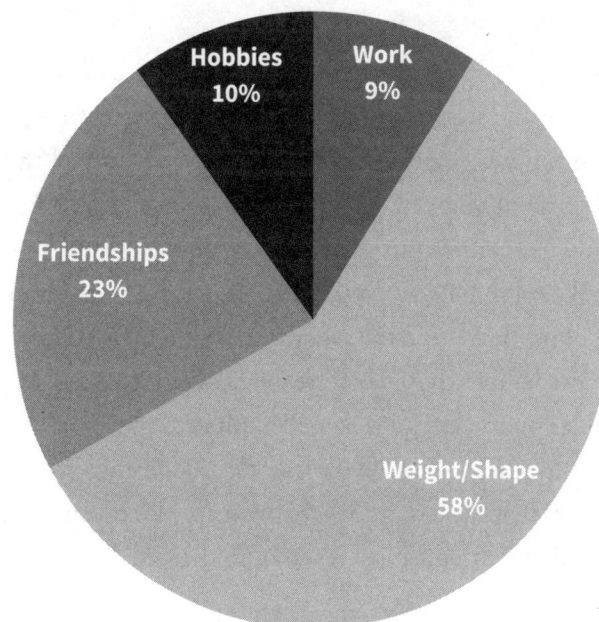

Hobbies 10%
Work 9%
Friendships 23%
Weight/Shape 58%

Maria started to think about how she wanted this pie chart to look a year from now. She considered things that have made her happy or given her a sense of accomplishment. She considered what connected her to her friends, family, and community. She made a list of these different areas and created a new pie chart for the future.

Maria's Pie Chart for the Future

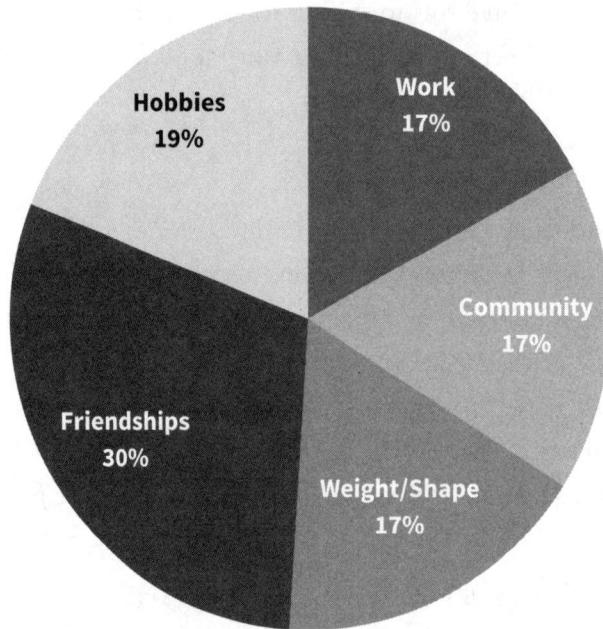

You might notice that shape and weight are still listed on Maria's future pie chart, which is okay. Realistically, this may still be a part of how you think about yourself and the time and energy you spend on different areas throughout your day. The key is to consider how balanced you feel among these different domains. If you notice that things are out of balance, think about how you can reduce time spent in one area to make room for the things that are most important to you.

You might be wondering, how do I figure out what is most important to me? How do I know what to include in this pie chart? Remember that everyone's pie chart looks different. Some people find it helpful to examine their values more closely to consider what to include. Values are a way to think about what is most important to you in your life. Rather than focusing on goals or accomplishments —the *what*—focusing on values helps you consider the ways in which you want to live your life—the *how*. For example, when considering friendships, you might identify that you want to be a supportive and trustworthy friend. It doesn't matter how many friends you have or how often you get to see them—you can strive for support and trustworthiness regardless.

Some people also like to review lists of values to help them determine what fits best for them. We have provided a link to a sample list in the online resources.

Exploring Your Self-Worth

Below are key areas that frequently shape self-worth. These may not all be relevant to you; add any others that are important.

1. Family

2. Friendships and social networks

3. Health and well-being

4. Recreation and hobbies

5. Creativity

6. Work, education, volunteering

7. Community involvement, liberation, justice

8. Shape, weight, and your ability to control them

9. _____

10. _____

11. _____

1. Once you have considered your values and areas of your life, draw your current pie chart depicting how you spend your time and energy.

My Pie Chart Currently

2. How does your current pie chart align with important areas and values? Are there areas that seem unbalanced?

_____

_____

_____

_____

_____

3. How much space does your control of shape and weight occupy? Did this surprise you? Has this changed over time?

_____

_____

_____

4. To which areas would you like to devote less time or resources?

_____

_____

_____

5. To which areas would you like to dedicate more time? Are there activities you have enjoyed that you would like to add?

_____

_____

_____

_____

6. What are some practical ways to minimize the time you spend in areas you would like to de-emphasize?

_____

_____

_____

_____

7. After considering these questions, create your desired pie chart for the future. Think about an ideal balance that you would like to strive for. Keep in mind that shape and weight may still play a role in your self-worth, and that's okay.

My Pie Chart for the Future

8. What is one change you can make this week to move in the direction of your desired pie chart? This could be a reduction of activities in one domain or adding time or resources in another.

_____

_____

_____

9. What potential barriers may arise, and how can you address them?

_____

_____

_____

_____

Challenging Your Thoughts

Most people have many automatic thoughts running through their minds and pay little attention to them. Some of these thoughts can contribute to feelings and eating disorder behaviors. You may discover that when you've had a negative experience with a particular situation, your thoughts about the situation have a greater influence on your experience than the situation itself.

For example, let's say you pass your coworker in the hallway. Rather than greeting you, they don't catch your eye and walk right by. What comes to mind? Do you think, "Why didn't he smile at me?" "He must be mad at me" or "What did I do to upset him?" Does it impact how you feel or behave toward him?

_____

_____

Now imagine the same situation but consider an alternative thought: "I know he has a hectic schedule today and I know he gets very focused when he's stressed." How would you feel if you had this thought instead? How would you behave?

_____

_____

As you can see, in precisely the same situation, your interpretation of your coworker's behavior—the thoughts in your head—influenced how you felt, and perhaps in turn how you behaved.

Let's look back at one of the times you restricted, binged, overexercised, purged, or engaged in some other eating disorder behavior. Just before the behavior, what did you say to yourself?

_____

_____

_____

These thoughts could include messages like:

- I know I'll be eating more later, so I should eat less now.

- Since I already blew my diet, I might as well just finish the package and start my diet again tomorrow.

- I ate too much—I need to get it out of my body so I don't gain weight.

If you had unhelpful thoughts like the ones above, you have a chance to challenge their truth. Below, we'll give you a tool to help you reframe unhelpful thoughts so they cause less harm and leave room for other possibilities. First, we will share an example to walk you through this process, and then provide a blank template (also available online) for you to complete.

- *Abraham's Story*

    Abraham had more cookies than he planned after dinner one night and decided to eat the rest of the package before bed. He identified that before his binge, he had the thoughts, "I've already eaten more than I intended, so I might as well finish the cookies even though I feel sick. Then I can start eating better tomorrow."

Reframing Unhelpful Thoughts, Abraham's Example

What is the thought you want to challenge?

I've already eaten more than I intended, so I might as well finish the cookies even though I feel sick. Then I can start eating better tomorrow.

Is this thought a statement of truth?   ☐ Yes   ☑ No

What is the evidence that supports this thought?

Well I did eat more than I intended and it made me feel uncomfortable.

What is the evidence against it? (Think as if you are a lawyer and focus on facts.)

Just because I have eaten more doesn't mean that I have to deprive myself of cookies tomorrow.

What are the consequences of that thought? Assuming it was true, what happened next?

Finishing the cookies and depriving myself tomorrow just maintains the cycle of my disordered eating.

What are alternative ways of thinking about that situation? Assuming these alternative interpretations, how would the consequences change?

I can stop now and accept that I ate more cookies than I intended. I don't have to finish them tonight or start a new diet tomorrow. The cookies will be there for me when I want them.

Reframing Unhelpful Thoughts

What is the thought you want to challenge?

_____

_____

Is this thought a statement of truth?   ☐ Yes   ☐ No

What is the evidence that supports this thought?

_____

_____

_____

What is the evidence against it? (Think as if you are a lawyer and focus on facts.)

_____

_____

_____

What are the consequences of that thought? Assuming it was true, what happened next?

_____

_____

_____

_____

What are alternative ways of thinking about that situation? Assuming these alternative interpretations, how would the consequences change?

_____

_____

_____

_____

You may need to use the worksheets to remember the prompts initially, but with practice you will notice it happening more automatically. If you struggle to reframe your thoughts, another strategy is to create mental distance from them. Try to notice the thought without judgment and neutralize it. Say to yourself, "I am having the thought that I should skip breakfast after eating the cookies last night. That is just a thought, and I don't have to do it. I can watch the thought float away." We want to emphasize that you do not need to thought-challenge your way out of experiences of discrimination or mistreatment, and there may be times when these strategies are useful.

Eating Disorder Mindsets

People with disordered eating often experience a mindset that filters the way they interpret information and drives their behaviors. For example, some people will experience a restriction mindset where they have urges to eat less. We like to think of mindsets as apps on your phones. Whenever your eating disorder gets activated, the app opens. You can train yourself to close the app. Eating disorder thoughts such as "I should lose weight" or "What is the lower calorie option on the menu?" may still arise. In our thin-focused society, expecting these thoughts to disappear entirely is unrealistic. But you can avoid opening the apps. They may run in the background and drain your battery slightly, but you can tune them out. As you progress in recovery, you may notice that you spend less time in the eating disorder mindset.

Core Beliefs

Automatic thoughts, described previously, occupy the surface level—they are the most accessible and easiest to identify. Core beliefs, on the other hand, are deeper-held beliefs that organize our thoughts and experiences (Greenberger and Padesky 2016). Core beliefs are usually absolute statements about ourselves, others, or the world. Common core beliefs among people with disordered eating are:

- I'm worthless.

- I'm unlovable.

- I must be perfect.

- I must be thin to deserve love.

- I'm not good enough.

If you can relate to some of the beliefs above, you can explore this further using the online resource Core Beliefs. The following worksheet, which is also online, will help you delve into this process.

Challenging Core Beliefs

What is the core belief that you would like to change?

_____

_____

How much do you believe this core belief? (0 to 100 percent) _____

What is the alternative or opposite core belief you would like to work toward?

_____

_____

How much do you believe this alternative core belief? (0 to 100 percent) _____

Collect evidence in support of the alternative core belief.

_____

_____

_____

_____

_____

Continue collecting evidence until you are able to increase your belief in your alternative core belief to at least 50 percent. Remember that this process may take several weeks or even months!

_____

_____

_____

_____

_____

Once you have strengthened your belief in your first alternative belief, consider whether there are other core beliefs you would like to change. These could be related to your disordered eating symptoms or more general core beliefs that may have an impact on your overall self-esteem. Repeat the process above to develop an alternative belief and gather evidence to strengthen this over time.

_____

_____

_____

_____

_____

Perfectionism

Perfectionism puts people at risk of developing and maintaining disordered eating (Stackpole et al. 2023). People who struggle with perfectionism often don't identify with it because they believe that to experience it, they must meet their "perfect" standard—and when you struggle with perfectionism, you're never going to meet that standard.

Take a moment to reflect on the characteristics of perfectionism below. Check off anything that applies to you. Are there any characteristics that you would add to the list?

Thoughts

☐ I must do everything well.

☐ I must do things right the first time.

☐ Nothing I do is done well enough.

☐ If I'm not the best, I'm the worst.

☐ Outside of my achievements or accomplishments, nothing (or very little else) matters.

☐ I focus mostly on criticism—what hasn't been achieved or done well—and discount praise for the positive things that I've done.

☐ _____

☐ _____

Behaviors

☐ Procrastination or putting things off until the last minute because of fear that you won't do them well.

☐ Checking and rechecking things—like assignments, work projects, appearance—and comparing them to others' performance or another standard.

☐ Not letting anyone's innocent mistakes—or your own—"slide."

☐ Avoidance of activities, tasks, or jobs where you might "fail."

☐ Avoidance of performance assessment.

☐ Discounting or downplaying your successes—that is, failing to "savor" any accomplishments because you're always striving toward the next one.

☐ _____

☐ _____

Accompanying Emotions

☐ Anxiety

☐ Stress and irritability

☐ Guilt

☐ Depression

☐ _____

☐ _____

In which areas of life—if any—do you aim to be perfect? Examples may include your work, relationships, appearance, sports, or health behaviors.

_____

_____

_____

What are the "rules" that you have for yourself in these areas? *Hint:* Sometimes these aims might start with "I must" or "I should":

- "I must be financially successful."

- "I have to do all of my scheduled workouts for the week."

- "I should appear to be happy and be kind all of the time."

- _____

- _____

- _____

- _____

Who has asked you to do (or be) the things you described above?

_____

_____

_____

What Fuels Perfectionism?

You may wonder whether it is possible to be perfect—spoiler alert: the answer is no—and if there is truly anything wrong with being a perfectionist. Perfectionism is a component of dominant culture, and perfectionistic behaviors may develop as a protection from other larger forces at play—such as discrimination, productivity expectations, or trauma. As Hilary Kinavey and Dana Sturtevant write in their 2022 book *Reclaiming Body Trust*, "Perfectionism is a protective flex when we can't tolerate our own humanity and we live in dehumanizing systems." Often, perfectionism is maintained by the behavioral process of reinforcement or reward. This process can trap us in a cycle of never-ending striving and expectations.

• *Zola's Story*

Zola's family moved to the United States from Iran when she was twelve. She remembered feeling overwhelmed with changes and recalled teasing and ridicule from her peers as she struggled to fit in. Around this time, she remembered pouring herself into her studies and spending hours on homework, double-checking, and sometimes even triple-checking assignments to ensure that her grammar was correct or to avoid "careless" mistakes.

Before coming to the United States, her teachers in Iran commented that she would occasionally omit words in her written work and fail to check her work fully. They also noticed that she had trouble communicating her needs and often seemed distracted. She told herself that she would be the "best" student in class and was praised by her new teachers for the work she completed. As she progressed through high school, she participated in several different clubs and activities to get into a top-tier college. She took on progressively larger leadership roles at school and became active in track and field. She remembered thinking, "If I'm going to do something, I should be the best at it."

Despite her activities and time spent on homework, she never felt like she could "keep it together" and often felt disorganized and scattered. Her anxiety about academics and doing well in school led her to begin procrastinating on homework. Around this time, she started to cope with anxiety by binge eating in the evenings, which led to her restricting during the following school days.

While in college, she had discussions with her therapist about the lifelong struggles with inattention and communication that drove her perfectionistic behaviors and thoughts. An educational psychologist diagnosed Zola with a language processing disorder and ADHD. She realized that for her, perfectionism acted as a way to overcome her then-undiagnosed challenges with neurodivergence.

Traditional CBT has labeled perfectionism as "psychopathology" and asks people to stop or reduce their perfectionistic behaviors. These include behaviors like checking things multiple times, avoidance behaviors, excessive organizing or list-making, and reading and speaking slowly to avoid mistakes.

We'd like to note that for many, perfectionistic thoughts and behaviors become a survival tactic and a way to keep afloat in a cutthroat, capitalist society. This is especially true for people assigned female at birth, fat folks, individuals with disabilities, and BIPOC people. Marginalized people often *do* have to work harder to get the same treatment or outcome as someone with more advantages and resources. This reality may be further confirmed when the person is faced with unfair treatment and inequity. Use the following worksheet to explore your experience with perfectionism. This worksheet and another one, Changing Perfectionistic Beliefs and Behaviors, are both available online.

Challenging Perfectionism

Do you notice a tendency toward perfectionism or striving for very high standards? When did this start? What was happening at the time?

_____

_____

_____

_____

In what ways does perfectionism and striving keep your disordered eating going? How, if at all, are these connected?

_____

_____

_____

_____

Some perfectionistic behaviors may have been helpful. Take a moment to reflect on anything that your perfectionistic beliefs or behaviors have given you. In what ways might they have served a function or helped you in the past? What are the advantages to holding these beliefs and performing these behaviors?

_____

_____

_____

_____

What are the costs of striving to achieve and "be perfect"? How realistic is it to continue to do this in the long run? What consequences might you experience?

_____

_____

_____

How might life look different if you aimed for average work instead of stellar work? What do you believe prevents you from allowing yourself to be "average"?

_____

_____

If you hold marginalized identities, are there real potential impacts to making these changes?

_____

_____

We want to name the feeling of being overwhelmed that might arise when examining and challenging perfectionism. Instead of getting critical about your perfectionism, get curious about how and when it might be showing up and whether your current behaviors are working for or against you. We also acknowledge that certain recommendations offered here may not be accessible to everyone at all times. Be compassionate toward yourself as you consider the next steps in the journey toward healing your relationship with food and your body.

Do you remember when you challenged your food rules in chapter 6? Challenging perfectionism is very similar to breaking food rules. We invite you to apply this process to any current rules that you have surrounding your performance or other areas of life outside of eating. If it feels accessible, complete the following activity over the next week.

What is the perfectionistic behavior that you are considering changing?

_____

What is one step you can take to change the behavior?

_____

Once you make changes, what are some things you notice?

_____

Summary of Takeaways

Chapter 8 covered self-esteem and how it ties into core beliefs and perfectionism. Here are some of the points covered in this chapter:

- Self-esteem can be tied to how we spend our time and energy in different areas of our lives. We discussed how to consider balance among these different life areas.

- Thoughts and beliefs about ourselves also contribute significantly to our self-esteem and can maintain eating disorders.

- Perfectionism is often connected to beliefs that impact self-esteem, and we discussed ways to change perfectionistic thoughts and behaviors.

Reflection

What did you find most helpful in chapter 8? What have you learned about your self-esteem and values? Reflect on aspects of this chapter you would like to remember as you continue the workbook. Self-esteem is a vast topic that can be a great area to explore with your therapist or support system.

_____

_____

_____

_____

_____

_____

When to Move on to Chapter 9

- You have completed your current and future pie charts, identified values in different life domains, and thought about how you can work toward shifting balance among the different areas of your life.

- You have considered the role of core beliefs and perfectionism in terms of self-esteem and thought about ways to modify unhelpful core beliefs and address perfectionistic thoughts and behaviors.

Chapter 9

Standing Up to Diet Culture

Now that you have explored your body image, self-esteem, and core beliefs, you better understand how diet culture has impacted these areas. You may be wondering, what do I do next? How do I move forward in a world where diet culture dominates? This chapter will offer suggestions for effectively navigating these challenges. First, let's check in again with your progress over the last week. Take a few moments to review your self-monitoring record from last week and complete the following tracker (also available online).

Weekly Progress Tracker 5

	Day 1	Day 2	Day 3	Day 4	Day 5	Day 6	Day 7
Eating Routines							
Ate breakfast							
Ate lunch							
Ate dinner							
Ate snacks							
Ate every 2–4 hours							
Ate a variety of foods							

	Day 1	Day 2	Day 3	Day 4	Day 5	Day 6	Day 7
Meals kept me feeling satisfied							
Enjoyed the food I was eating							
Other Eating Behaviors							
Restriction							
Binge eating							
Self-induced vomiting							
Laxative use							
Excessive exercise or movement							
Excessive water or caffeine							
Body checking							
Body avoidance							
Other behaviors (e.g., chewing and spitting, using saunas, etc.)							

What are you noticing about your progress this week?

_____

_____

_____

Assertive Communication

Assertive communication is a style of communication that allows you to express yourself clearly and directly, advocate for your needs, and defend your boundaries while also respecting the needs and opinions of others. Initially, this may feel challenging, especially if you tend to be more passive. However, over time, this communication style can help you feel more confident, improve self-esteem, improve relationships, and help you effectively meet your needs. Some assertive communication strategies include:

- Use "I" messages to help communicate your feelings while minimizing defensive reactions in others. For example, "I feel annoyed when you don't help me clean up the dishes after dinner."

- State your point of view or request clearly. For example, "I would like you to plan our next date night."

- Share facts about the situation rather than relying on judgment or interpretation. "I have noticed that you didn't respond to my text messages, and I've felt neglected."

- Try to ensure that nonverbal communication is also assertive. Speak at your usual volume, maintain eye contact if that feels comfortable for you, and use relaxed body language.

Assertiveness looks different for everyone. What is considered "confident" in one culture may feel unsafe or inappropriate in another. Keep in mind that assertive communication takes practice. Consider in which situations you may want to practice these skills. And each time you do, allow yourself to reflect and process what you've learned. Use the following worksheet (also available online) to help you.

Practicing Assertive Communication

In which situations might more assertive communication be helpful for you?

_____

_____

_____

When you think about communicating assertively, what worries come to mind?

_____

_____

_____

How can you help yourself prepare or practice for more assertive communication?

_____

_____

Practice using the four steps to write out a script regarding this situation:

1. Use "I" statement to communicate your feelings:

    _____

2. State your point of view or request clearly:

    _____

    _____

3. Share facts about the situation without judgment:

    _____

    _____

    _____

4. Identify nonverbal strategies to help convey your message:

    _____

    _____

Assertive communication can also help when you encounter diet culture or pressure to change your shape or weight. Remember that you may not feel ready to have these conversations with others—and there's nothing wrong with that. For many with disordered eating, it can take time to feel comfortable standing up to these expectations. Sometimes, direct confrontation or communication may not feel safe or accessible. In any case, you'll also probably need to set boundaries with others.

Setting Boundaries

As you become aware of how diet culture affects your day-to-day life, you may start to notice more comments and behaviors from friends, family, and health care providers that impact you. One thing to keep in mind: Diet culture is everywhere.

Setting Boundaries with Family, Friends, and Peers

The people with whom you interact daily have likely experienced many of the same pressures you have, and they may be at different points in their relationship with food and body. Rather than focusing on changing their opinion or how they feel about themselves, try to focus on your needs in the relationship. Consider some of the following strategies.

Situation	Suggested Responses
Someone engaging in diet talk	"I would rather not discuss diets or weight loss." "I would like to spend our time catching up rather than focusing on dieting or food." "I'm trying not to think about foods as good or bad, and it has been helping me a lot." Casually change the subject.
Someone making negative comments about their body or others' bodies	"I prefer not to make negative comments about my body." "I've been trying not to comment about other people's appearance." "I don't feel comfortable talking about this. Can we talk about something else?"
Someone commenting on your weight or body	"I prefer that people do not comment on my body." "I am trying to move away from discussing changes in my body and weight."

Situation	Suggested Responses
Someone commenting that they are concerned about your health	"I appreciate your concern, but I do not feel comfortable discussing this with you." "My health is my business, and we do not need to discuss it." "This is not an appropriate time to discuss this."

When you prepare to set boundaries with friends and family, it is important to gauge how much emotional energy you have for these conversations. You may not feel ready to be assertive in all situations or with all the people in your life. That's okay—even ignoring a comment or casually changing the subject can be a good starting point to change your interactions with others. Take it slow, and think about how you can find support from other friends, family members, or community members you trust. Keep in mind that setting boundaries can include internal decisions and nonverbal limits too.

Setting Boundaries with Health Care Providers

As we discussed earlier, health care providers are a common source of weight bias. Requesting care and attending medical appointments can create stress for people with disordered eating. Consider also the power differential in these relationships as well as your safety. For some in larger bodies and with other marginalized identities, challenging providers can result in being labeled as "uncooperative" or "combative," with potentially devastating consequences. The control health care providers wield over access to certain treatments and medications can add to the anxiety about using assertive communication when accessing health care. The following strategies may be a good starting point, but it may be helpful to weigh the pros and cons of using these tools with your health care providers.

Situation	Suggested Responses
You would prefer not to be weighed at appointments.	"I would prefer not to be weighed today." "Please let the doctor know that I prefer not to be weighed, and I am happy to discuss it more in our appointment." "Can you explain why my weight is necessary for today's appointment? I would prefer not to step on the scale unless it is needed."

Situation	Suggested Responses
Weight is brought up by the doctor when your visit is about an unrelated problem.	"I would like to focus on the issue that I requested this appointment for instead of my weight." "I would prefer not to discuss my weight today."
A diet or weight loss treatment is recommended without a prior discussion or request.	"I am not interested in a diet or weight loss treatment at this time." "I am working to improve my relationship with food. I will let you know if I need any more assistance in this area."
Weight loss is recommended over another treatment that was requested.	"Is this the same treatment you would recommend for someone in a smaller body?" "Can you share the research with me that supports weight loss instead of the treatment I have requested?"

As we noted in the section on friends and family above, always consider your emotional energy and the safety you feel in having these conversations. Remember to give yourself the option to disengage from these conversations if you are feeling unsafe or threatened, especially if you are a part of a marginalized community. Seek support from friends, family members, and community members if you need assistance in advocating for yourself.

Finding Community

Throughout this workbook, you've learned individual strategies to help you improve your relationship with food and your body. You've spent time and mental energy unlearning and challenging many deeply held belief systems. Some perspectives introduced in this book are *countercultural*, meaning that they go against the mainstream beliefs of society. We live in a culture that considers it desirable and virtuous to maintain a low weight, to overexercise, to restrict calories, and to deny ourselves tasty food. It's no wonder recovery from an eating disorder feels unattainable when society has its own healing to do!

The swim upstream can be lonely if you lack company. For many, the path to recovery includes both individual healing and community building. Genuine communication, emotional vulnerability, and collective challenging of societal norms contribute to powerful shared experiences that can cement recovery. A sense of belonging can combat loneliness and isolation—two experiences that often work in tandem to maintain eating disorders. Connections with friends, health care providers, recovering peers, colleagues, religious communities, and other external support systems can be key factors in recovery from disordered eating (Leonidas and dos Santos 2014; Wolfe et al. 2024).

If you struggle to build close social connections or to find community, you're not alone. As a society, we increasingly spend more time alone (Atalay 2024). Eating disorders thrive in isolation. Isolation and disordered eating become a vicious cycle. Even after you've recovered from your eating disorder, you might find that the years you spent stuck in it took you away from others. You might have also interacted with people or groups who made recovery difficult. Below we offer a list of ideas for finding people or a community that can support your recovery.

- Check out clubs or groups based on interests outside of the eating disorder.

- Volunteer.

- Try apps to meet new people (Meetup or Bumble BFF).

- Explore new hobbies.

- Join a book club.

- Rekindle a friendship by texting or calling an old friend.

- Attend networking events.

- Learn a new skill or trade.

- Take a class in the community.

In some areas, finding an in-person recovery community that understands your needs and supports body diversity may be difficult. If this is the case, virtual environments with pro-recovery messaging may provide the support you need. Consider finding online communities through weight-inclusive providers and social media. For those who may not be interested in forging relationships based on eating disorder recovery, there are other resources. Listening to podcasts, subscribing to digital newsletters, or curating your social media feed can help reinforce the messages you learned here. Check our online resources for more ideas. Commit to spending fifteen minutes listening to a podcast or reading something from one of our resources.

If you are in a larger body, finding others who also navigate the world in a larger body can be especially helpful. If you have no people in your physical community, then our resources can help you create your own virtual network. A network like this can be valuable for connecting you with resources for self-care, shopping, and advocacy. It may feel this way now, but you are not the only person facing this challenge. Use the following worksheet (also available online) to think about building community.

Building Community

Who provides you with social support?

_____

_____

If you have limited social support right now, has there been a time in your life when you have had closer connections? What helped you to foster connections?

_____

_____

How does your support system influence your eating disorder recovery? What's helpful? What remains challenging?

_____

_____

_____

_____

Are there any ideas listed above that you'd be interested in trying?

_____

_____

Are there social media resources or podcasts you'd like to check out? Take a moment to find them now.

_____

_____

If building a community feels overwhelming, take a breath and offer yourself kindness. Creating community can take time and energy that isn't always readily available. If necessary, come back to this section when you feel ready.

Summary of Takeaways

Chapter 9 covered assertive communication and how to use these strategies to set boundaries with friends, family members, and health care providers. We also discussed how to build a community for additional support. Here are the main takeaways:

- Assertive communication can help you meet your needs and set boundaries in your relationships.

- These communication strategies can help you stand up for yourself in challenging situations.

- Many people notice that finding and building community can be valuable throughout their recovery.

Reflection

What did you find most helpful in chapter 9? In what areas can you imagine using assertive communication strategies? Would it help to use these techniques with friends, family members, or your health care team?

_____

_____

_____

_____

_____

When to Move on to Chapter 10

- You have completed the reflection exercises and considered how you would like to use these communication strategies.

- You have considered a plan to build community in your life if desired.

Chapter 10

Relapse Prevention

Congratulations on making it to chapter 10! You have put in the effort and persevered, and that should be celebrated. In this final chapter we will review your progress and help you create a plan for maintaining the changes you've made. Remember: Recovery is a process, and it is not usually linear. Setbacks should be expected, but with the use of the skills you've gained, you can help yourself move forward.

Review of Progress

Let's review the eating disorder signs you identified in chapter 1 and see whether any have changed or improved. You can also look back at your weekly progress trackers and see what trends you notice.

Eating Disorder Signs	Experiencing Now	Improved?
I think about my eating, weight, or shape frequently.		
Food dominates my life.		
I am preoccupied with a desire to change my body—to lose weight, to become more muscular, etc.		
I try to restrict how much food I eat most of the time.		
I try to follow strict rules about what I eat, how much I eat, and when I eat.		

Eating Disorder Signs	Experiencing Now	Improved?
I try to stay within a certain number of calories during the day.		
I refuse to eat certain types of food.		
I have rituals related to eating, such as eating certain foods first or chewing a certain number of times.		
I feel a loss of control when eating; it's hard to stop once I've started.		
I am compelled to eat things I believe I should not eat.		
I often feel the desire to eat when emotionally upset or stressed.		
I feel guilty after eating.		
I find myself "grazing" or snacking frequently throughout the day.		
I eat unusually large amounts of food in a short period of time.		
I make myself vomit to lose weight or after eating a large amount of food.		
I use laxatives, diuretics, or diet pills to lose weight or after eating large amounts of food.		
I use water, caffeinated beverages, or nicotine to stay full during the day.		
I use exercise to make up for eating large amounts of food.		
I force myself to exercise even if I am tired, injured, or do not feel like exercising.		
I feel guilty if I skip a workout or take a day off from exercise.		
I need to track my exercise and/or how many calories I burn during the day.		
I try to avoid eating in front of other people.		
I frequently check my weight, appearance in the mirror, or how my clothes fit.		
I frequently compare myself to others or to pictures of myself.		

Eating Disorder Signs	Experiencing Now	Improved?
I feel very distressed about my body appearance, weight, and/or shape.		
I try to avoid looking at my body and/or avoid other people seeing my body.		
My sense of self-worth is closely tied to my feelings about my weight, shape, and body.		

Use the following worksheet (also available online) to reflect on your progress.

Progress Review

In which areas have you progressed?

_____

_____

_____

Which areas do you still struggle with?

_____

_____

_____

What, if any, changes have you made to your behavior to better align with your values?

_____

_____

Which strategies from this workbook can you use to keep addressing the behaviors you would still like to address?

_____

_____

Do you need any additional support? Reflect on your needs below.

_____

_____

Tapering Off Self-Monitoring

If you have progressed with eating more regularly and have experienced a reduction in the eating disorder behaviors above, now it's time to phase out self-monitoring. Remember when we told you we didn't expect you to do this forever? You can always return to self-monitoring if you hit another rough patch. Many people find that self-monitoring alone is a great strategy for getting back on track when they've had a resurgence of symptoms or a lapse.

Maintaining Progress

Recovery from an eating disorder takes time. You did not develop your eating disorder overnight, and it usually won't go away quickly. It is important to remember that no one can recover perfectly, and there may be slips and relapses during recovery. This is to be expected.

Lapse vs. Relapse

It might be helpful to consider the difference between a *lapse* and a *relapse*. A lapse might be defined as a setback or the return of some symptoms, but short of a full return of your disordered eating. A relapse is a return to more severe symptoms. Think of a lapse as tripping while climbing up a mountain, whereas a relapse may involve sliding down to the mountain's base to where you started.

The following Relapse Prevention Plan (also available online) may help prevent a lapse from becoming a relapse.

Relapse Prevention Plan

Part 1: Useful Strategies

List the behaviors and strategies useful to you in your recovery so far. Go through the earlier chapters of this workbook and see which skills have been most helpful to you. You might include in your list some of the following: self-monitoring, meal planning, regular eating, alternative coping strategies, harm reduction strategies, self-compassion, eating more food, incorporating avoided foods, challenging body checking or avoidance, body appreciation, and so on.

My List of Recovery Behaviors and Strategies

1. _____

2. _____

3. _____

4. _____

5. _____

6. _____

7. _____

8. _____

9. _____

10. _____

Part 2: High-Risk Situations

Next, try to anticipate the high-risk situations you are likely to encounter that could increase the risk of slips and relapses. Below are some things you may want to include on your list:

- Stress or a busy schedule, which makes planning meals difficult

- Becoming overwhelmed by feelings and emotions

- Loss of a family member or friend

- Marital, social, or family problems

- Change in schedule, such as going on summer break, moving, or going away to school

- Changes in weight

- Friends or family members dieting

- Missing a meal or snack

- Experiencing discrimination or oppression

- Being told by a medical professional to lose weight or change your diet

- Receiving a new medical diagnosis

- Being in unfamiliar food environments or ones with unrestricted access to food, such as a buffet, holiday meal, or potluck

- Having limited access to food

- Getting weighed at the doctor's office

- Shopping for clothes

- Pregnancy

- Dating

- Others commenting on your weight

- Events where your appearance may be more noticeable, such as weddings, graduations, or religious ceremonies

My List of High-Risk Situations

1. _____

2. _____

3. _____

4. _____

5. _____

6. _____

7. _____

8. _____

9. _____

10. _____

Part 3: Early Warning Signs

Become familiar with the early warning signs of a relapse. Potential early warning signs might include any of your previous eating disorder symptoms. You might want to review the list of signs of eating disorders earlier in the chapter. Examples may include weight loss, skipping meals, or bingeing. Once you've identified a warning sign, assign a coping strategy that can help you address it.

Warning Sign	Coping Strategy
I noticed myself skipping breakfast again	Regular eating and meal planning

Part 4: Cope Ahead

In times of crisis, you may find it difficult to remember healthy coping methods. Many people in crisis resort to familiar ways of coping. Making a plan ahead of time can help break these patterns of behavior. Make a list of ten things you can do instead of reverting to eating disorder behaviors to cope. After the list is completed, keep it in a place where it can be accessed—your refrigerator, cupboard, or even a screenshot on your phone. You can also refer to the list of alternative coping strategies in chapter 5.

My List of Crisis Coping Strategies

1. _____

2. _____

3. _____

4. _____

5. _____

6. _____

7. _____

8. _____

9. _____

10. _____

Where will you keep this list?

_____

Part 5: Enlisting Supports

It is also important to reach out during crises—or when you feel scared, alone, or out of control. Talking about your feelings can relieve some of your anxiety and help prevent a slip or relapse. Reaching out also helps remind you that you are not alone. Use the space below to write down the names of people you can rely on for support. Asking for help may make you feel vulnerable, but the more you do it, the easier it will become.

My List of Social Support

1. _____

2. _____

3. _____

4. _____

5. _____

6. _____

7. _____

8. _____

9. _____

10. _____

What do you think will be most important in terms of maintaining progress? What are the helpful elements of your relapse prevention plan?

_____

_____

_____

_____

_____

Next Steps and When to Seek Help Again

- Once you have finished your final review of symptoms and completed your relapse prevention plan, consider reviewing any of the online resources that you have not had time to explore.

- Keep your relapse prevention plan somewhere you can easily access it when you need it.

- Continue exploring the books, podcasts, and other resources provided throughout the workbook and in the online materials. There are some great options to support the hard work you have completed!

During recovery, slips and relapses are common. Many people tend to be hard on themselves if they have a slip or relapse. Remember that no recovery is perfect. If you have a bad day, forgive yourself, put it behind you, and continue to move forward in your recovery. It is important to look back at the lapse to learn from it and simultaneously be compassionate. Instead of looking at a lapse as a failure, think of it as an opportunity to identify skills that you can use in the future.

Congratulations!

As you near the end of the book, we hope you can take a moment to congratulate yourself on the time, thought, and energy you've invested in completing this workbook. Wherever you may be in your journey, know that you've taken meaningful steps forward. Revisit this workbook at any time to remind yourself of your progress. We hope that you are empowered to stand up to diet culture and feel better equipped to nourish and support yourself during hard times. We wish you all the best in your recovery and beyond.

Summary of Takeaways

In chapter 10, we reviewed your overall progress in this treatment by considering:

- Which symptoms have improved and the ones you would like to continue to address.

- Stopping self-monitoring and reincorporating it as needed.

- What a lapse looks like and how to use your Relapse Prevention Plan when you notice setbacks.

- When to seek help again in the future.

References

Academy for Eating Disorders. 2021. *Eating Disorders: A Guide to Medical Care.* 4th ed. Wakefield, MA: Academy for Eating Disorders.

Academy for Eating Disorders. 2015. "Nine Truths About Eating Disorders." https://www.aedweb.org/resources/publications/nine-truths.

Atalay, E. 2024. "A Twenty-First Century of Solitude? Time Alone and Together in the United States." *Journal of Population Economics* 37 (1).

Ayton, A., and A. Ibrahim. 2018. "Does UK Medical Education Provide Doctors with Sufficient Skills and Knowledge to Manage Patients with Eating Disorders Safely?" *Postgraduate Medical Journal* 94 (1113): 374–80.

Barakat, S., S. A. McLean, E. Bryant, A. Le, P. Marks, S. Touyz, and S. Maguire. 2023. "Risk Factors for Eating Disorders: Findings from a Rapid Review." *Journal of Eating Disorders* 11 (1): 1–31.

Bartel, S., S. L. McElroy, D. Levangie, and A. Keshen. 2024. "Use of Glucagon-like Peptide-1 Receptor Agonists in Eating Disorder Populations." *International Journal of Eating Disorders* 57 (2): 286–93.

Becker, C. B., K. M. Middlemass, F. Gomez, and A. Martinez-Abrego. 2019. "Eating Disorder Pathology Among Individuals Living with Food Insecurity: A Replication Study." *Clinical Psychological Science* 7 (5): 1144–58.

Bennett, W. 1983. *Dieter's Dilemma.* New York: Basic Books.

Brandenburg, B. M. P., and A. E. Andersen. 2007. "Unintentional Onset of Anorexia Nervosa." *Eating and Weight Disorders: Studies on Anorexia, Bulimia, and Obesity* 12 (2): 97–100.

Brown, T. A., P. Klimek-Johnson, J. A. Siegel, A. D. Convertino, V. J. Douglas, J. Pachankis, and A. J. Blashill. 2024. "Promoting Resilience to Improve Disordered Eating (PRIDE): A Case Series of an Eating Disorder Treatment for Sexual Minority Individuals." *International Journal of Eating Disorders* 57 (3).

Brownstone, L. M., and A. M. Bardone-Cone. 2021. "Subjective Binge Eating: A Marker of Disordered Eating and Broader Psychological Distress." *Eating and Weight Disorders: Studies on Anorexia, Bulimia, and Obesity* 26 (7): 2201–9.

Burke, N. L., V. M. Hazzard, L. M. Schaefer, M. Simone, J. L. O'Flynn, and R. F. Rodgers. 2023. "Socioeconomic Status and Eating Disorder Prevalence: At the Intersections of Gender Identity, Sexual Orientation, and Race/Ethnicity." *Psychological Medicine* 53 (9): 1–11.

Butler, R. M., and R. G. Heimberg. 2020. "Exposure Therapy for Eating Disorders: A Systematic Review." *Clinical Psychology Review* 78 (1): 101851.

Butler, R. M., and C. A. Levinson. 2024. "Addressing Body Dissatisfaction in Women in Larger Bodies Using Exposure-Based Interventions: A Case Report." *Clinical Case Studies* 23 (6): 419–31.

Byrne, S. M, and A. Fursland. 2024. "New Understandings Meet Old Treatments: Putting a Contemporary Face on Established Protocols." *Journal of Eating Disorders* 12 (1).

Cash, T. 2008. *The Body Image Workbook*. Oakland, CA: New Harbinger Publications.

Centers for Disease Control and Prevention. 2024. "Social Determinants of Health." https://www.cdc.gov/about/priorities/social-determinants-of-health-at-cdc.html?CDC_AAref_Val=https://www.cdc.gov/about/sdoh/index.htm.

Chastain, R. 2022. "Reader Question: What's the Difference Between Weight-Neutral Health and Weight-Inclusive Health?" Substack.com, August 27. https://weightandhealthcare.substack.com/p/reader-question-whats-the-difference-acb.

Christian, C., and C. A. Levinson. 2022. "An Integrated Review of Fear and Avoidance Learning in Anxiety Disorders and Application to Eating Disorders." *New Ideas in Psychology* 67 (December): 100964.

Cobbaert, L., and A. Rose. 2023. *Eating Disorders and Neurodivergence: A Stepped Care Approach.* Sydney, Australia: Eating Disorders Neurodiversity Australia.

Conason, A. 2021. *The Diet-Free Revolution*. Berkeley, CA: North Atlantic Books.

Conceição, E. M., L. M. Utzinger, and E. M. Pisetsky. 2015. "Eating Disorders and Problematic Eating Behaviours Before and After Bariatric Surgery: Characterization, Assessment, and Association with Treatment Outcomes." *European Eating Disorders Review* 23 (6): 417–25.

Craighead, L. W. 2006. *The Appetite Awareness Workbook*. Oakland, CA: New Harbinger Publications.

Diemer, E. W., J. M. W. Hughto, A. R. Gordon, C. Guss, S. B. Austin, and S. L. Reisner. 2018. "Beyond the Binary: Differences in Eating Disorder Prevalence by Gender Identity in a Transgender Sample." *Transgender Health* 3 (1): 17–23.

Duncan, A. E., H. N. Ziobrowski, and G. Nicol. 2017. "The Prevalence of Past 12-Month and Lifetime DSM-IV Eating Disorders by BMI Category in US Men and Women." *European Eating Disorders Review* 25 (3): 165–71.

Eddy, K. T., D. J. Dorer, D. L. Franko, K. Tahilani, H. Thompson-Brenner, and D. B. Herzog. 2008. "Diagnostic Crossover in Anorexia Nervosa and Bulimia Nervosa: Implications for *DSM-V*." *American Journal of Psychiatry* 165 (2): 245–50.

Eisenberg, M. E., A. Carlson-McGuire, S. E. Gollust, and D. Neumark-Sztainer. 2014. "A Content Analysis of Weight Stigmatization in Popular Television Programming for Adolescents." *International Journal of Eating Disorders* 48 (6): 759–66.

Ellison, J. M., H. K. Simonich, S. A. Wonderlich, R. D. Crosby, L. Cao, J. E. Mitchell, T. L. Smith, M. H. Klein, S. J. Crow, and C. B. Peterson. 2016. "Meal Patterning in the Treatment of Bulimia Nervosa." *Eating Behaviors* 20 (January): 39–42.

Fairburn, C. G. 2008. *Cognitive Behavior Therapy and Eating Disorders*. New York: Guilford Press.

Fairburn, C. G., S. Bailey-Straebler, S. Basden, H. A. Doll, R. Jones, R. Murphy, M. E. O'Connor, and Z. Cooper. 2015. "A Transdiagnostic Comparison of Enhanced Cognitive Behaviour Therapy (CBT-E) and Interpersonal Psychotherapy in the Treatment of Eating Disorders." *Behaviour Research and Therapy* 70 (July): 64–71.

Flegal, K. M. 2023. "Use and Misuse of BMI Categories." AMA *Journal of Ethics* 25 (7): 550–58.

Flint, S. W., M. Čadek, S. C. Codreanu, V. Ivić, C. Zomer, and A. Gomoiu. 2016. "Obesity Discrimination in the Recruitment Process: 'You're Not Hired!'" *Frontiers in Psychology* 7 (647).

Froreich, F. V., S. E. Ratcliffe, and L. R. Vartanian. 2020. "Blind Versus Open Weighing from an Eating Disorder Patient Perspective." *Journal of Eating Disorders* 8 (39).

Gaudiani, J. L. 2019. *Sick Enough: A Guide to the Medical Complications of Eating Disorders*. New York: Routledge.

Golden, N. H. 2023. "Atypical Anorexia Nervosa Is Not Atypical at All! Commentary on Walsh et al. (2022)." *International Journal of Eating Disorders* 56 (4).

Golden, N. H., and P. S. Mehler. 2020. "Atypical Anorexia Nervosa Can Be Just as Bad." *Cleveland Clinic Journal of Medicine* 87 (3): 172–74.

Gordon, A. 2020. *What We Don't Talk About When We Talk About Fat*. Boston: Beacon Press.

Greenberger, D., and C. A. Padesky. 2016. *Mind over Mood: Change How You Feel by Changing the Way You Think*. 2nd ed. New York: Guilford Press.

Harrison, D. 2021. *Belly of the Beast: The Politics of Anti-Fatness as Anti-Blackness*. Berkeley, CA: North Atlantic Books.

Hart, K. E., and P. Chiovari. 1998. "Inhibition of Eating Behavior: Negative Cognitive Effects of Dieting." *Journal of Clinical Psychology* 54 (4): 427–30.

Hazzard, V. M., K. A. Loth, L. Hooper, and C. B. Becker. 2020. "Food Insecurity and Eating Disorders: A Review of Emerging Evidence." *Current Psychiatry Reports* 22 (12).

Jakubek, K. 2023. "AMA Adopts New Policy Clarifying Role of BMI as a Measure in Medicine." American Medical Association. https://www.ama-assn.org/press-center/press-releases/ ama-adopts-new-policy-clarifying-role-bmi-measure-medicine.

Kater, K. 2012. *Healthy Bodies: Teaching Kids What They Need to Know*. North St. Paul, MN: Body Image Health.

Keel, P. K., L. P. Bodell, A. A. Haedt-Matt, D. L. Williams, and J. Appelbaum. 2017. "Weight Suppression and Bulimic Syndrome Maintenance: Preliminary Findings for the Mediating Role of Leptin." *International Journal of Eating Disorders* 50 (12): 1432–36.

Kesby, A., S. Maguire, R. Brownlow, and J. R. Grisham. 2017. "Intolerance of Uncertainty in Eating Disorders: An Update on the Field." *Clinical Psychology Review* 56 (August): 94–105.

Keys, A. 1950. *The Biology of Human Starvation*. London: Geoffrey Cumberlege.

Kinavey, H., and D. Sturtevant. 2022. *Reclaiming Body Trust*. New York: Penguin.

Kinavey, H., and D. Sturtevant. 2024. "Body Trust Tuesday." *Center for Body Trust Newsletter.* https://centerforbodytrust.com/newsletters.

Lawrence, S. E., R. M. Puhl, M. B. Schwartz, R. J. Watson, and G. D. Foster. 2022. "'The Most Hurtful Thing I've Ever Experienced': A Qualitative Examination of the Nature of Experiences of Weight Stigma by Family Members." *SSM: Qualitative Research in Health* 2: 100073.

Lawrence, S. E., R. M. Puhl, R. J. Watson, M. B. Schwartz, L. M. Lessard, and G. D. Foster. 2023. "Family-Based Weight Stigma and Psychosocial Health: A Multinational Comparison." *Obesity* 31 (6): 1666–77.

Lazzer, S., F. Agosti, P. Silvestri, H. Derumeaux-Burel, and A. Sartorio. 2007. "Prediction of Resting Energy Expenditure in Severely Obese Italian Women." *Journal of Endocrinological Investigation* 30 (1): 20–27.

Leonidas, C., and M. A. dos Santos. 2014. "Social Support Networks and Eating Disorders: An Integrative Review of the Literature." *Neuropsychiatric Disease and Treatment* 10 (May): 915.

Levinson, C. A., L. Fewell, and L. C. Brosof. 2017. "My Fitness Pal Calorie Tracker Usage in the Eating Disorders." *Eating Behaviors* 27: 14–16.

Levinson, C. A., H. F. Fitterman-Harris, S. Patterson, E. Harrop, C. Turner, M. May, D. Steinberg, L. Muhlheim, R. Millner, E. Trujillo-ChiVacuan, J. Averyt, R. Peebles, S. Rosenbluth, and C. B. Becker. 2023. "The Unintentional Harms of Weight Management Treatment: Time for a Change." *The Behavior Therapist* 46 (7): 271–82.

Li, P., X. Chen, and Q. Yao. 2021. "Body Mass and Income: Gender and Occupational Differences." *International Journal of Environmental Research and Public Health* 18 (18): 9599.

Linardon, J., Z. McClure, T. L. Tylka, and M. Fuller-Tyszkiewicz. 2022. "Body Appreciation and Its Psychological Correlates: A Systematic Review and Meta-Analysis." *Body Image* 42 (September): 287–96.

Linardon, J., and M. Messer. 2019. "My Fitness Pal Usage in Men: Associations with Eating Disorder Symptoms and Psychosocial Impairment." *Eating Behaviors* 33 (April): 13–17.

McEntee, M. L., S. R. Philip, and S. M. Phelan. 2023. "Dismantling Weight Stigma in Eating Disorder Treatment: Next Steps for the Field." *Frontiers in Psychiatry* 14.

Morgan-Lowes, K. L., C. Thøgersen-Ntoumani, J. Howell, V. Khossousi, and S. J. Egan. 2023. "Self-Compassion and Clinical Eating Disorder Symptoms: A Systematic Review." *Clinical Psychologist* 27 (3): 269–83.

Mueller, D., E. Bacalso, A. Ortega-Williams, D. J. Pate, and J. Topitzes. 2021. "A Mutual Process of Healing Self and Healing the Community: A Qualitative Study of Coping with and Healing from Stress, Adversity, and Trauma Among Diverse Residents of a Midwestern City." *Journal of Community Psychology* 49 (5).

Nagata, J. M., C. D. Otmar, C. M. Lee, E. J. Compte, J. M. Lavender, T. A. Brown, K. T. Forbush, A. Flentje, M. E. Lubensky, J. Obedin-Maliver, and R. L. Mitchell. 2025. "Community Norms of the Eating Pathology Symptoms Inventory (EPSI) in Cisgender Sexual Minority Adults." *Eating and Weight Disorders: Studies on Anorexia, Bulimia, and Obesity* 30 (1).

Neel, J. 1962. "Diabetes Mellitus: A 'Thrifty' Genotype Rendered Detrimental by 'Progress'?" *American Journal of Human Genetics* 14 (4): 353.

Neff, K., and C. K. Germer. 2018. *The Mindful Self-Compassion Workbook: A Proven Way to Accept Yourself, Build Inner Strength, and Thrive.* New York: Guilford Press.

Parker, L. L., and J. A. Harriger. 2020. "Eating Disorders and Disordered Eating Behaviors in the LGBT Population: A Review of the Literature." *Journal of Eating Disorders* 8 (1).

Pinciotti, C. M., Z. Smith, S. Singh, C. T. Wetterneck, and M. T. Williams. 2022. "Call to Action: Recommendations for Justice-Based Treatment of Obsessive-Compulsive Disorder with Sexual Orientation and Gender Themes." *Behavior Therapy* 53 (2): 153–69.

Puhl, R. M., T. Andreyeva, and K. D. Brownell. 2008. "Perceptions of Weight Discrimination: Prevalence and Comparison to Race and Gender Discrimination in America." *International Journal of Obesity* 32 (6): 992–1000.

Puhl, R., and Y. Suh. 2015. "Health Consequences of Weight Stigma: Implications for Obesity Prevention and Treatment." *Current Obesity Reports* 4 (2): 182–90.

Ramaswamy, N., and N. Ramaswamy. 2023. "Overreliance on BMI and Delayed Care for Patients with Higher BMI and Disordered Eating." *AMA Journal of Ethics* 25 (7): E540–44.

Robbins, M., K. Rinaldi, P. M. Brochu, and J. L. Mensinger. 2025. "Words Are Heavy: Weight-Related Terminology Preferences Are Associated with Larger-Bodied People's Health Behaviors and Beliefs." *Body Image* 53: 101860.

Rodin, J., L. Silberstein, and R. S. Moore. 1984. "Women and Weight: A Normative Discontent." *Nebraska Symposium on Motivation* 32 (November): 266–308.

Santoniccolo, F., and L. Rollè. 2024. "The Role of Minority Stress in Disordered Eating: A Systematic Review of the Literature." *Eating and Weight Disorders: Studies on Anorexia, Bulimia, and Obesity* 29 (1).

Schröder, S. S., U. N. Danner, A. A. Spek, and A. A. van Elburg. 2022. "Problematic Eating Behaviours of Autistic Women: A Scoping Review." *European Eating Disorders Review* 30 (5): 510–37.

Sivyer, K., E. Allen, Z. Cooper, S. Bailey-Straebler, M. E. O'Connor, C. G. Fairburn, and R. Murphy. 2020. "Mediators of Change in Cognitive Behavior Therapy and Interpersonal Psychotherapy for Eating Disorders: A Secondary Analysis of a Transdiagnostic Randomized Controlled Trial." *International Journal of Eating Disorders* 53 (12).

Sonneville, K. R., and S. K. Lipson. 2018. "Disparities in Eating Disorder Diagnosis and Treatment According to Weight Status, Race/Ethnicity, Socioeconomic Background, and Sex Among College Students." *International Journal of Eating Disorders* 51 (6): 518–26.

Srivastava, P., A. Giannone, E. W. Lampe, O. M. Clancy, B. Fitzpatrick, A. S. Juarascio, and S. M. Manasse. 2024. "A Naturalistic Examination of Feeling Fat: Characteristics, Predictors, and the Relationship with Eating Disorder Behaviors." *International Journal of Eating Disorders* 57 (8): 1756–68.

Stackpole, R., D. Greene, E. Bills, and S. J. Egan. 2023. "The Association Between Eating Disorders and Perfectionism in Adults: A Systematic Review and Meta-Analysis." *Eating Behaviors* 50 (August): 101769.

Sterling, W., and C. Crosbie. 2023. *How to Nourish Yourself Through an Eating Disorder*. New York: The Experiment.

Stice, E., J. M. Gau, P. Rohde, and H. Shaw. 2017. "Risk Factors That Predict Future Onset of Each DSM-5 Eating Disorder: Predictive Specificity in High-Risk Adolescent Females." *Journal of Abnormal Psychology* 126 (1): 38–51.

Strings, S. 2019. *Fearing the Black Body: The Racial Origins of Fat Phobia*. New York: New York University Press.

Tantleff-Dunn, S., R. D. Barnes, and J. G. Larose. 2011. "It's Not Just a 'Woman Thing': The Current State of Normative Discontent." *Eating Disorders* 19 (5): 392–402.

Taylor, S. R. 2021. *The Body Is Not an Apology: The Power of Radical Self-Love*. Oakland, CA: Berrett-Koehler Publishers.

Tomiyama, A. J., D. Carr, E. M. Granberg, B. Major, E. Robinson, A. R. Sutin, and A. Brewis. 2018. "How and Why Weight Stigma Drives the Obesity 'Epidemic' and Harms Health." *BMC Medicine* 16 (1).

Trottier, K., and D. E. MacDonald. 2017. "Update on Psychological Trauma, Other Severe Adverse Experiences, and Eating Disorders: State of the Research and Future Research Directions." *Current Psychiatry Reports* 19 (8).

Tovar, V. 2018. *You Have the Right to Remain Fat*. New York: The Feminist Press at CUNY.

Tylka, T. L., and N. L. Wood-Barcalow. 2015a. "The Body Appreciation Scale-2: Item Refinement and Psychometric Evaluation." *Body Image* 12 (1): 53–67.

Tylka, T. L., and N. L. Wood-Barcalow. 2015b. "What Is and What Is Not Positive Body Image? Conceptual Foundations and Construct Definition." *Body Image* 14 (14): 118–29.

Vadiveloo, M., and J. Mattei. 2017. "Perceived Weight Discrimination and 10-Year Risk of Allostatic Load Among US Adults." *Annals of Behavioral Medicine* 51 (1): 94–104.

Wolfe, H., C. B. Shepherd, R. G. Boswell, J. Genet, and W. Oliver-Pyatt. 2024. "Discovering a 'Sense of Community': Patient Experiences of Connection in Intentionally Remote Eating Disorder Care." *Journal of Eating Disorders* 12 (1).

Wood-Barcalow, N., T. L. Tylka, and C. Judge. 2021. *Positive Body Image Workbook: A Clinical and Self-Improvement Guide*. Cambridge, UK: Cambridge University Press.

Yao, S., R. Kuja-Halkola, J. Martin, Y. Lu, P. Lichtenstein, C. Norring, A. Birgegård, Z. Yilmaz, C. Hübel, H. Watson, J. Baker, and C. Almqvist. 2019. "Associations Between Attention-Deficit/ Hyperactivity Disorder and Various Eating Disorders: A Swedish Nationwide Population Study Using Multiple Genetically Informative Approaches." *Biological Psychiatry* 86 (8): 577–86.

Yilmaz, Z., A. Hardaway, and C. Bulik. 2015. "Genetics and Epigenetics of Eating Disorders." *Advances in Genomics and Genetics* 5 (March): 131–50.

Lauren Muhlheim, PsyD, is a psychologist, fellow of the Academy for Eating Disorders (AED), certified eating disorder specialist (CEDS), and approved consultant for the International Association of Eating Disorder Professionals (IAEDP). Muhlheim is also a Certified Body Trust Provider (CBTP). She directs Eating Disorder Therapy LA, a group practice in Los Angeles, CA. She is certified in family-based treatment (FBT) for adolescent eating disorders, and is author of *When Your Teen Has an Eating Disorder.*

Muhlheim has held leadership roles in several professional organizations, including the AED, IAEDP, and the Los Angeles County Psychological Association. She has previously been an IAEDP core course instructor. She provides training on eating disorders to mental health providers and parents internationally. She has a website and a blog, and has built a solid professional platform around weight-inclusive modified evidence-based treatments for eating disorders, specifically, cognitive behavioral therapy (CBT) and FBT.

Jennifer Averyt, PhD, ABPP, is a board-certified clinical health psychologist based in Phoenix, AZ. She provides weight-inclusive care for individuals with eating disorders and chronic health concerns, as well as training and consultation in the delivery of evidence-based eating disorder treatment.

Shannon Patterson, MEd, PhD, is a licensed psychologist based in Madison, WI, with a specialized focus on the intersection of eating disorder treatment and psychological adjustment to chronic illness. She is founder and owner of a private practice, offering both in-person and virtual therapy to individuals across the United States. Beyond her direct care services, Shannon holds an educational role at an eating disorder treatment company where she provides training and consultation to therapists and health care professionals across the United States. She also contributes to the advancement of the field as an ad hoc reviewer for the *International Journal of Eating Disorders.*

Foreword writer **Carolyn Black Becker, PhD,** is professor of psychology at Trinity University and a licensed, board-certified clinical psychologist who specializes in the treatment and research of eating disorders, PTSD, and anxiety-based disorders.

Real change *is* possible

For more than fifty years, New Harbinger has published proven-effective self-help books and pioneering workbooks to help readers of all ages and backgrounds improve mental health and well-being, and achieve lasting personal growth. In addition, our spirituality books offer profound guidance for deepening awareness and cultivating healing, self-discovery, and fulfillment.

Founded by psychologist Matthew McKay and Patrick Fanning, New Harbinger is proud to be an independent, employee-owned company. Our books reflect our core values of integrity, innovation, commitment, sustainability, compassion, and trust. Written by leaders in the field and recommended by therapists worldwide, New Harbinger books are practical, accessible, and provide real tools for real change.

newharbingerpublications

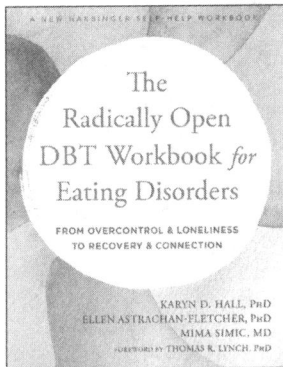

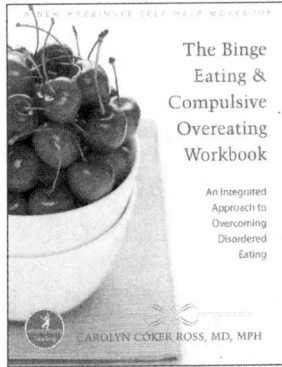

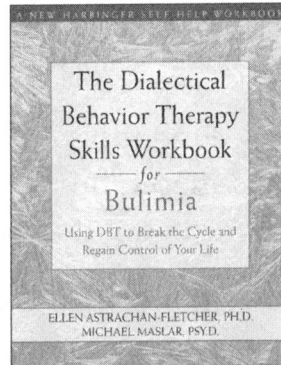

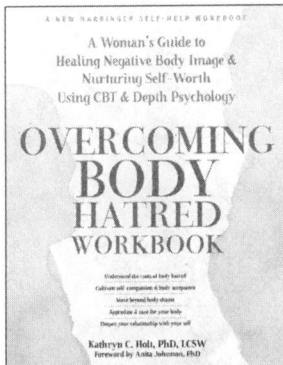

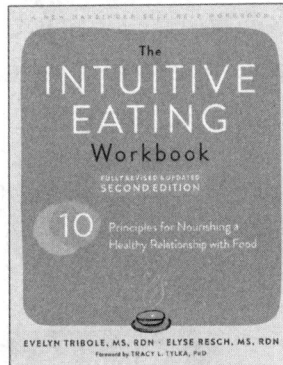

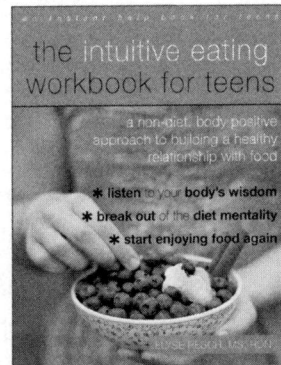

Did you know there are **free tools** you can download for this book?

Free tools are things like **worksheets, guided meditation exercises,** and **more** that will help you get the most out of your book.

You can download free tools for this book—whether you bought or borrowed it, in any format, from any source—from the New Harbinger website. All you need is a NewHarbinger.com account. Just use the URL provided in this book to view the free tools that are available for it. Then, click on the "download" button for the free tool you want, and follow the prompts that appear to log in to your NewHarbinger.com account and download the material.

You can also save the free tools for this book to your **Free Tools Library** so you can access them again anytime, just by logging in to your account! Just look for this button on the book's free tools page.

+ Save this to my free tools library

If you need help accessing or downloading free tools, visit **newharbinger.com/faq** or contact us at **customerservice@newharbinger.com.**